Transcultural Nursing

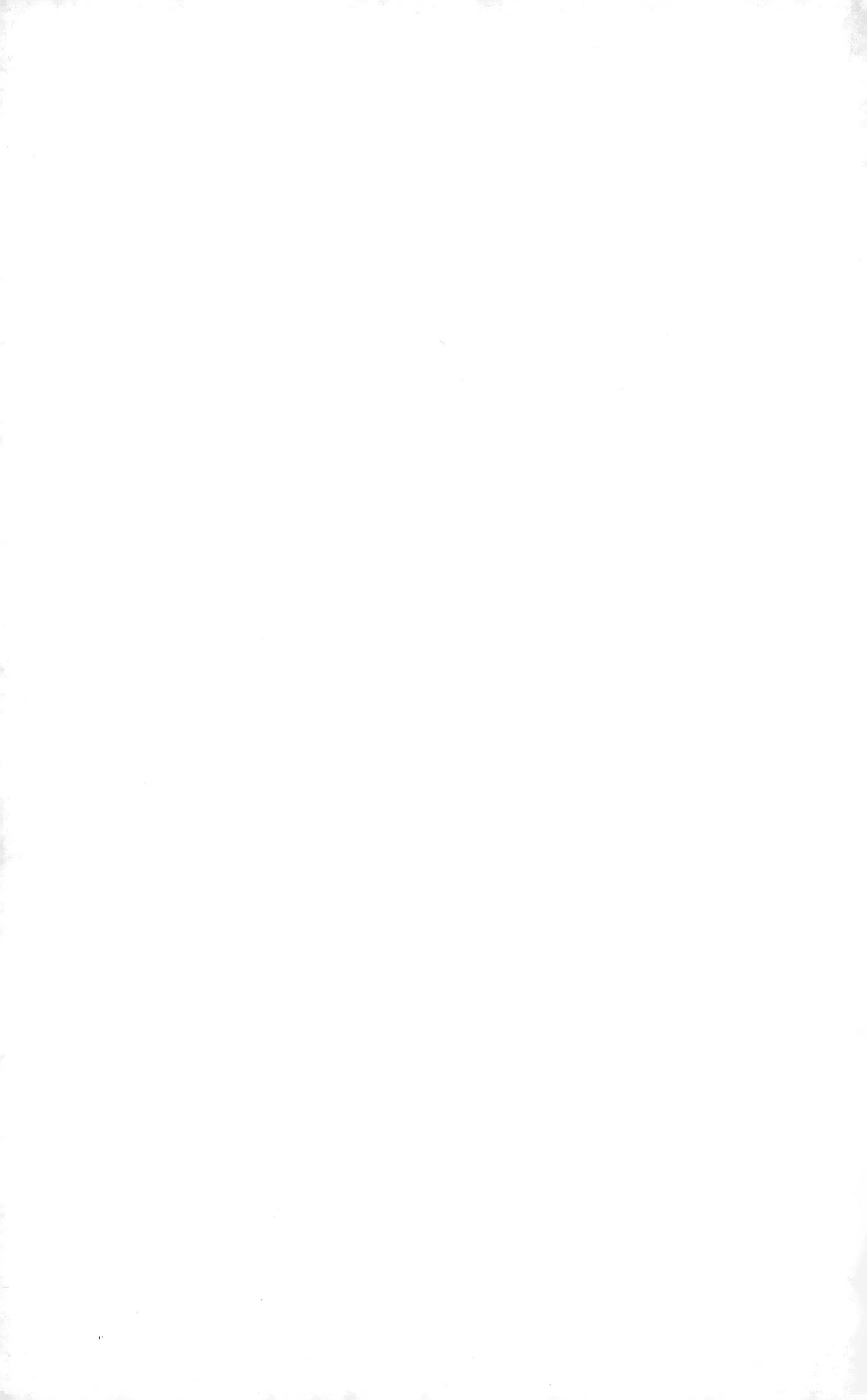

Transcultural Nursing

A BOOK OF READINGS

Edited By
PAMELA J. BRINK
University of Alberta, Edmonton

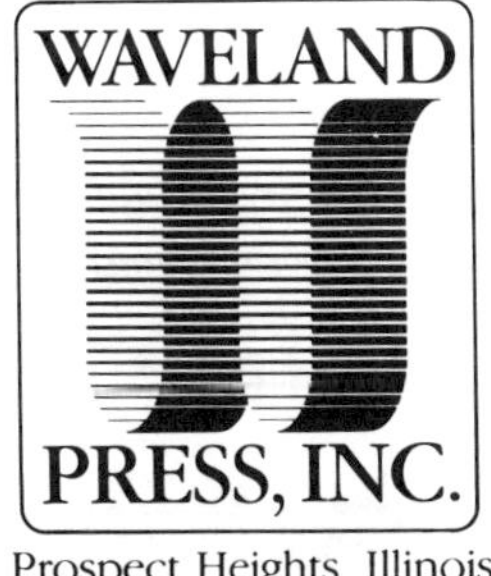

Prospect Heights, Illinois

For information about this book, write or call:
Waveland Press, Inc.
P.O. Box 400
Prospect Heights, Illinois 60070
(708) 634-0081

1990 reissued by Waveland Press, Inc.

ISBN 0-88133-486-3

Printed in the United States of America

7 6 5 4 3 2

Contents

Preface

Nursing, as a profession, has become increasingly aware of the cultural differences in patients. With this awareness has come a greater demand for literature on various cultural and subcultural groups. The need for more and more information cannot be met, totally, through the nursing journals, so nurses are faced with the problem of having to discover the significance of cultural differences for themselves. How can one set about this process of discovery? Not every nurse can go back to school to get a doctorate in medical anthropology, nor would the profession be served through this means. Not every nurse can go out and "do field work" in some distant country in order to experience the rigors of transcultural research. Instead, most nurses will contact people individually and experience, on a personal level, transcultural nursing. This book is intended for the practitioner, in whatever setting, who is interested in patients from other cultures.

This collection of readings from nurses, nurse-anthropologists, and anthropologists deal with some cultural differences among peoples. This is not a "how to do it" book, but rather is intended to raise the cultural consciousness of the reader. The themes around which the articles are grouped involve interdigitation between nursing and applied anthropology. Articles discuss cultural differences in relation to child rearing, language, value systems, personality, and research methods.

Pamela J. Brink

Transcultural Nursing

Introduction

Transcultural Nursing was created through the blend of the fields of anthropology and nursing. The field began with nurses doing their doctoral research in anthropology and returning to nursing. They, in turn, taught the theories and methods of anthropology they saw as most relevant and applicable to nursing. It was Madeleine Leininger who gave the new field its name, Transcultural Nursing. The original points of contact were in the areas of social and cultural anthropology, physical anthropology, and linguistics. Today, nurses may major in Transcultural Nursing. As its name implies, transcultural nursing is nursing that transcends cultural boundaries seeking to find the essence of nursing that applies in all cultural contexts. Transcultural nursing is concerned with comparative communications systems, comparative anatomy and physiology, and comparative cultural norms within health care. Like every other branch of nursing, transcultural nursing is concerned with the nurse-patient relationship, the nursing process, the health care delivery system, nursing education, and nursing administration, but it approaches the art and science of nursing from the cultural perspective.

Transcultural (or cross-cultural) nursing is the fusion of nursing and anthropology in both theory and practice. Nursing theory has always been concerned with the nurse and the patient/client, both separately and in interaction. Nursing practice occurs within a variety of settings, with goals for primary, secondary and tertiary prevention. Nursing is an active profession; it does things to, for, and with people. As such, nursing's interest lies with the human being—whether ill or well—within a multitude of contexts. Unlike medicine, physiology or chemistry, nursing lays no claim to a specific area of knowledge which can be clearly defined or circumscribed. Nursing knowledge is an accumulation and synthesis of knowledge derived from widely diverse fields, all of which relate in some way to nursing care. Nursing is a very pragmatic profession which acquires information for its usability. Anything which may have remote or immediate applicability to the practice of nursing becomes nursing content.

Fundamentally, nursing is concerned with human behavior, whether that behavior is associated with the patient/client, the nurse, other health professionals, or anyone else the nurse may contact in the performance of nursing. Whatever affects human behavior eventually affects nursing. For this reason, nursing involves itself with the physical sciences such as chemistry, physics and biology, since these fields are concerned with the basic parameters within which human life occurs. Other areas, equally important, include history, philosophy and the arts. The social sciences—psychology, sociology, anthropology—increase nursing's awareness of human emotions, motivations, social organization, and belief systems. Each art and science has developed theories and methods to discover and explain the usual and the aberrant; the normal and the abnormal; the average and the deviant. The nurse is expected to have a basic understanding of the norms and deviations of the norm in the human as a bio-psycho-socio-cultural being.

Transcultural nursing, yields theories and methods applicable to both nursing and anthropology. Nursing uses the theories and methods of anthropology and applies them to nursing practice. The result is transcultural nursing. Nursing can translate its theories and practices into cultural contexts to share with anthropology; the result is the same. It is the clinical component that makes transcultural nursing, *nursing* and the cultural component of nursing practice that makes it *transcultural*; both components must be present.

The core of nursing is the nurse-patient relationship expressed in the nursing process. All areas of nursing, whether research, education, or administration, are all directly or indirectly impacted upon by assessment, diagnosis, intervention, and evaluation of patient care. The nursing process requires the basic dyad of the nurse and the patient/client. Nursing also occurs within health care delivery institutions or agencies which are composed of structures and people. These interrelationships of space, time and personnel are all culturally defined.

Transcultural nursing can be studied at many levels: as basic knowledge; as clinical practice or as theory building. This book has chosen to look at transcultural nursing from the perspective of the nursing process. It is a beginning reader in the field, and the articles chosen have aimed at breadth rather than depth. Each article was conceived of as an introduction to a particular aspect of nursing across cultural boundaries. Many more problems and issues exist than those included in that section, but each article discusses some aspect of the cultural variable that could be incorporated into a standard nursing assessment. The section "Methods and Strategies" emphasizes participant observation as an assessment method, since nursing uses this form of data collection regularly. "Integration through Application" associated specific groups with certain nursing problems but in no way exhausts the possible combinations that can occur.

The nursing process of assessment, diagnosis, intervention, and evaluation is heavily dependent upon the first step in the process—data collection. Yet what kind of data must be collected? How does the nurse know what information will be relevant? What is done with the data, once collected? These questions have been asked for decades and are not in the least new. When a nurse is told, "Be sure to assess for the cultural variable" what is the cultural variable? Kluckhohn and Mowrer speak of traditions, beliefs, and folklore as cultural determinants. What a person believes ultimately affects subsequent behavior. Florence Kluckhohn speaks of value orientations, or how people view their world and what is important to them. Benedict, on the other hand, says that the way people are raised affects their future behavior. Many of the problems nurses face can be directly traced to problems in intercultural communication. The list of cultural variables is an extensive one. All aspects of living have cultural components. The easiest definition to remember about culture, is that whatever a person believes to be true or right about any aspect of life, probably stems from culture.

If what a person believes is expressed in behavior, then one way to find out about a person's cultural background is to look and listen. Participant observation is the simplest means for collecting data for a nursing assessment. Talking to people, asking questions, observing what they do and when, are all part of the nursing process. The one added dimension in participant observation is to ask why. Byerly, Rosenhahn, and Ragucci all write about the method of participant observation. Byerly and Rosenhahn chose hospital settings, while Ragucci lived in an Italian-American neighborhood. The process is the same wherever the field worker goes. As a method, however, participant observation does have its limitations, as Myers humorously shows. The protection of human rights is always at risk in this form of data collection, but few research subjects object to this form of research. Indeed, most of us are ethnocentric, and believe that our culture is the best, so any individual who is interested in our culture is welcome.

Once the data has been collected, it must be organized into a meaningful package. The organization is dependent upon the purpose for which the data was collected. If the nurse is interested in knowing how to obtain a blood pressure reading, then the patient/client is asked about blood pressures. If the nurse is interested in follow-up care post partum, then ask questions about what the patient knows and believes about post partum follow-up.

The second phase of the nursing process, intervention, is totally dependent upon the findings. Foster states that the end result of applied anthropology is the achievement of specific kinds of changes in human behavior, whether in farming or in health habits. Nursing is predominantly interested in changing human behavior, either directly or indirectly, through nursing intervention. Teaching preventive or rehabilitation procedures is specifically aimed at changing the patient's behavior in relation to either health maintenance or health restoration. Much of direct patient care, particularly in community health and in psychiatric nursing, is aimed at change. In fact, the basic scale for evaluating nursing interventions is usually stated as "no change, minimal change, change in the predicted direction." Since both nursing and applied anthropology have as their goal change in human behavior for the purpose of improving the condition of the person being studied, then the model for applied anthropology as proposed by Foster should be easily adaptable to the nursing process.

If nurses, whatever their specialty, would view every patient care situation as a study sample of one, collect data on that case, and compare all cases at the end of a year's period, then generalizations could be made on the basis of that comparative data, and each nurse would have added to the body of nursing literature in that field. Nursing, like anthropology, is concerned with the totality of the subject under study, and has the advantage of being involved in participant observation daily. With such a wealth of data at their fingertips, nurses could easily contribute to the science of human behavior in a way that no other discipline can. Oliver Osborne speaks very cogently to the blending of nursing and anthropology to that end.

The articles by Foster and Osborne set the tone for this book since transcultural nursing is a blend of nursing and anthropology, but the nursing process is never complete without nursing interventions which are aimed at changing behavior. No one volume can possibly cover all of the published or unpublished works in a particular field, and so we must select those which appear most pertinent. Other articles and books relevant to the field of transcultural nursing are listed in each section. Further readings are provided through the lists of references associated with each article.

RECOMMENDED READINGS

Bauwens, Eleanor E., ed., *The Anthropology of Health*. St. Louis: The C.V. Mosby Company, 1978.

Branch, Marie F. and Phyllis P. Paxton, eds., *Providing Safe Nursing Care for Ethnic People of Color*. Englewood Cliffs, NJ: Prentice-Hall Inc., 1976.

Brink, Pamela J. "Key Issues in Nursing and Anthropology," in *Advances in Medical Social Science*, Vol. 2 (1984): 107-146. Julio L. Ruffini, ed., New York: Gordon and Breach Science Publishers.

Brownlee, Anne T., *Community, Culture, and Care: A Cross Cultural Guide to Health Care Workers*. St. Louis: The C.V. Mosby Company, 1978.

Clark, Anne L., ed., *Culture, Childbearing, Health Professionals*. Philadelphia: F.A. Davis Co., 1978.

Dougherty, Molly C. and Toni Tripp-Reimer, "The Interface of Nursing and Anthropology," *Annual Reviews of Anthropology* 14 (1985): 219-241.

Henderson, George and Martha Primeaux, *Transcultural Health Care*. Menlo Park, CA: Addison Wesley Publishing Company, 1981.

Leininger, Madeleine M., *Nursing and Anthropology: Two Worlds to Blend*. New York: John Wiley & Sons, Inc., 1970.

Leininger, Madeleine M., ed., *Transcultural Nursing: Concepts, Theories and Practices*. New York: John Wiley & Sons, Inc., 1978.

Orque, Modesta Soberano, Bobbie Block, and Lidia S. Ahumada Monrroy, *Ethnic Nursing Care: A Multicultural Approach*. St. Louis: The C.V. Mosby Company, 1983.

Spector, Rachel E., *Cultural Diversity in Health and Illness*. New York: Appleton Century Crofts, 1979.

Tripp-Reimer, Toni and Molly C. Dougherty, "Crosscultural Nursing Research," *Annual Review of Nursing Research* (1985): 77-104. Harriet H. Werley and Joyce J. Fitzpatrick, eds., New York: Springer Publishing Company.

Anthropology and Nursing: Some Common Traditions and Interests

OLIVER OSBORNE

Oliver Osborne raises the central issues involved in the blending of anthropology and nursing. He discusses the commonalities of both fields, the contributions each can make to the other in relation to knowledge or content, and the similarities in socialization in each field. For greater detail on the blend of nursing and anthropology the reader is directed to Madeleine Leininger's book, Nursing and Anthropology: Two Worlds to Blend, listed in the recommended readings in this section.

In the past two decades there has been an increasing approximation in the interests of social scientists and practitioners in the healing professions. Jaco suggests that the developing collaborations between social scientists and medical personnel result from the desire of practitioners of the healing arts to reconsider the extent of their biological bias and their atomistic, specializing approach to health care(1). Though the dominant theme today in medicine remains the particularistic, specializing emphasis, there is a developing literature which attends to the problems of "man" as an entity as well as "man" as he exists in his various ecological and sociocultural environments. This new medical definition of patients as "wholes" stems from an increasing, though not fully accepted, appreciation of the functional interdependence of the discrete organs which comprise man. This is to be contrasted with the earlier, and still prevalent, view of patients as compilations of diseased and normal organs. Jaco suggests that criticisms of the atomistic approach to medical practice stimulated medical practitioners to develop their conceptualizations of the wholeness of man.

An important aspect of this movement towards a more integrated conceptualization of man has been an attempt to effect closure between the mainstream of medical (bio-physiological) practitioners and those who treat disorders of the mind (psychiatrists). This reflects the medical practitioners attempts to breach the ancient western philosophical dichotomy of mind and matter, body and soul. The most apparent evidence of this movement has been the flowering of interest in the medical specialty of psychosomatic medicine.

Matarazzo suggests that this current concern with the patient as an entity, as contrasted with the concern with the condition of the organs of the patient has roots in earlier traditions of medical practice (2). He finds that the swing from specialization to comprehensive medical practice began as early as the 1930's. For him the roots of modern comprehensive medical practice are based upon an earlier custom of bedside medicine when the doctor made daily visits to their patients' homes. At that time important elements of medical care included understanding of the patient and supportive treatments.

The intensive and prolonged involvement of social scientists in the study of health care institutions has resulted in the development of groupings of these men who have accepted such identifications as medical sociologists and medical anthropologists. These people have created a nomenclature and a specialized body of literature suggestive of the problems and concerns peculiar to their new subdisciplines.

THE GENERALIZING NATURE OF ANTHROPOLOGY

Anthropology is frequently described as the "holistic study of man." The term "holistic" refers to the intellectual stance of anthropology. Bohannan in his introduction to his text, *Social Anthropology*, reaffirms the holistic tradition of anthropology.

> This book intends to instill immediately the stereo-scopic vision that is the hallmark of all successful anthropology and a necessity of the modern world(3).

Bohannan includes within his stereoscopic anthropological purview the studies of biology, sociology, personality, and culture. In the first chapter of their text, *An Introduction To Anthropology*, Beals and Hoijer elaborate the characteristics of this holistic tradition(4). They find that anthropology "is probably the most comprehensive of the sciences dealing with man and his works" for as a discipline anthropology approaches "both the biological and the social sciences."

In pursuit of its primary objective, "the study of man," anthropology has included as legitimate objects for study all of man's conditions and creations from the earliest times to the present. This means that anthropologists study man as a physical and psychological entity, as a social being, and as a creator and carrier of culture. Included among the various specialized areas within the general discipline of anthropology are cultural anthropology, social anthropology, culture and personality, physical anthropology, paleontology, archeology, and linguistics. Common to all of these separate anthropological studies is an interest in history and the problem of biological, social, and cultural change. To qualify as students of anthropology the workers in these areas must consider the study of man their primary concern. In his recent text, *Kinship and Marriage*, Robin Fox testifies to the centrality of the specification of "man" as the legitimate subject of anthropological studies. Although his book relates to the specialized and sophisticated study of kinship and marriage systems, an aspect of the larger anthropological interest in the comparative study of social systems, Fox acknowledges the "general aims" of anthropology:

> I am not particularly interested in the question "what is society?" but in what I take to be the truly anthropological question "what is Man?"(5)

Therefore, despite the fact of the vigorous and continuing investment of intellectual and physical energies in many specialized studies, the focus of the anthropologist remains "the study of man." In this respect anthropology is not only an holistic science, it is also a "generalizing" science.

MEDICAL ANTHROPOLOGY

Among the several studies which characterize anthropology some have had an intrinsic relationship to medical and nursing problems. This should not be surprising, for the highest and most comprehensive level of medical and nursing practice infers attempts to determine the correct pathological factors in man's physical and social environment, in man's psychology, as well as in man's organs.

Anthropological studies which have particular relevance to medical and nursing studies are physical anthropology, cultural anthropology, social anthropology, and culture and personality. It is the workers in these areas who have contributed the most to the study and the development of the literature in the area now known as medical anthropology. The general anthropological interest in problems of change is frequently interpreted, in medical anthropology, as the problem of the dissemination of health information and programs.

Physical anthropologists study evolutionary changes and population differences in the structure and function of the body. Hulse related physical anthropology to the medical tradition which he defines as concerned with "the desire to alleviate the suffering, and, if possible, cure the sick(6)." Compatible with the generalizing nature of anthropology Hulse finds that physical anthropology served to "unite the purely physical studies and the purely social studies of mankind."

Among the several studies in cultural anthropology there is an interest in ethnophysiology, ethnopsychology, ethnosociology, and cosmology. Findings in these areas suggest how people understand the functioning of their bodies and the natural and supernatural contexts in which their bodies are situated. These studies reveal the relationship between idea systems and behavior.

The social anthropologist is interested in the delineation and analysis of those patterns of social interaction which comprise social systems. Therefore, within the province of social anthropological concerns is the study of health institutions.

Study in the area of culture and personality expresses the anthropologists concern with the discernment of relationships between culture, social structure, and personality(7). In a more broadly conceived, holistic, anthropological tradition the basic determinants of personality are defined as nature or constitution (i.e., biology), society, and culture(8). Study in the area of culture and personality has contributed to our knowledge of physical, psychological, and social pathology. In fact, the most consistent and provocative studies in culture and personality have focused upon comparative studies of normal and abnormal behavior, comparative psychology, and, increasingly, comparative physiology.

THE GENERALIZING NATURE OF NURSING

In like manner, more completely than any other health profession, nursing has committed itself to the total care of the patient. The commitment of the nursing profession and nurses to total patient care parallels the anthropological tradition of the "holistic" study of man. This conceptualization of "total patient care" is a generalizing principle which gives form to nursing studies and nursing practice as the anthropological conceptualization of "the study of man" gives form and direction to anthropology.

The generalizing nature of nursing practice is no recent nursing innovation. Despite the fact that much ideology in nursing is based upon medical models the nature of nursing has never permitted nurses to create a nursing practice which parallels the segmented practice of the medical specialties. Despite the seeming exclusivity of the practice of public health nurses and psychiatric nurses, good nursing practice in these specialties must be based upon the generalizing imperative of total nursing care for total patient care. Recently, Cynthia H. Kelly provided an excellent example of this principle when she described how, during the 1967 Detroit uprising, public health nurses worked in hospitals during periods of regular nursing personnel shortages(9).

The literature suggests that the role of the clinical specialist infers improved ability to make efficacious referrals to a wide range of medical, social, and cultural institutions. The philosophy and programs of both undergraduate collegiate schools of nursing and two year community college schools of nursing will insure this generalizing tradition.

At this time it is not possible that the nurse will be able to specialize her practice to the same extent as the doctor. There is, in nursing, no parallel to the circumscribed, proprietary, and exclusive character of the doctor-patient relationship. With the exception of some aspects of military nursing, there is no nursing parallel to the superordinate-subordinate doctor-patient relationship.

It is the lack of these peculiarly exclusive, proprietary, and superordinate dimensions of the nurse's relationship to those subject to her care which creates the opportunity for the nurse to take into consideration the impact of her "self" and "others" upon her care of her patients. It is her appreciation of these factors which causes the nurse to pursue her investigations of the social and cultural systems in which her patient, a biological entity, exists. This is the "holistic" view of the patient. Thus, with good nursing care there is always a tendency towards generalized nursing care.

All of these considerations have contributed to the nursing professions development of a "stereoscopic" nursing practice similar, in many respects, to the "stereoscopic vision" which Bohannan considers to be the hallmark of anthropology(10).

THE ANTHROPOLOGICAL METHOD AND NURSING THEORY

It has been shown that there are many similarities between anthropological study and nursing practice. Both anthropology and nursing are holistic and generalizing in their study and practice.

Anthropology is also a descriptive and a comparative science. In their attempts to discover and define the "essence" of man anthropologists have developed the comparative study of physical, biological, psychological, social, and cultural systems. Essential to these comparisons is the adequacy of the descriptions which anthropologists construct from the phenomena they observe. The most difficult and continuing problem for the anthropologist remains the identification and construction of universal categories. Such universal categories are necessary for the proper ordering of data. They are prerequisite to efficacious cross cultural comparisons.

For nurses there remains the requirement of adequate descriptions of nursing practice. To date, such descriptions have been either too simplistic or prematurely problem oriented. Involved in this has been a tendency to describe patient-nurse interactions only as they illuminate certain constricted theoretical problems. There has also been too great a tendency to describe patient-nurse interactions only as the patient interacts with one institution or subdepartment of one institution. There is a need for more comprehensive patient care studies. Such studies should be diachronic as well as synchronic. The collection and comparison of such studies will reveal regularities in the patient-nurse relationship which will facilitate the development of general and efficient theories of nursing practice. The anthropological ethnography can be used as the prototype for descriptions of such interactions. In anthropology the ethnographic descriptions of social and cultural phenomena have contributed to the development of much anthropological theory within a short period of time.

There is, then, a need for nurses to consider the comparative approach to the development of nursing science and theory. There is, also, an equally important need for nurses to get more deeply involved in the study of nursing practice in other cultures. These are times of rapid social change and much seeking for understanding of the future directions of nursing contributions. Cross-cultural studies of nursing practice will provide depth and perspective to attempts to develop and enrich nursing competencies.

Intellectually we often dichotomize between underdeveloped nonwestern countries and developed western countries. The principal criterion for this judgment has been technological development. Sophistication in interpersonal relations, complex cosmologies, and highly developed arts have not been considered as equally important contributions to the definition of development. It is precisely in these less technological areas that cross-cultural nursing studies will contribute to our understanding of our patients as psychological, social, and cultural beings. Such studies will also contribute to our increased effectiveness in the organization and presentation of nursing services to the variety of publics which comprise the complex western community.

There are also benefits to be derived from study of the manner in which developing countries assimilate western technology. The interesting and important modifications which occur in such assimilations might be suggestive for the development of our own utilizations. Increased interest in the study of cross-cultural health problems suggests a possibility for future collaborations between the nurse and the anthropologist.

NURSING METHOD AND ANTHROPOLOGICAL THEORY

There are dimensions of the nursing method which are of value to the anthropologist. The nursing profession has committed itself to the belief that self-knowledge and understanding as well as the understanding and appreciation of the behaviors of others is an essential predicate of good nursing care. Since the early writing of Malinowski, anthropologists have understood the value of this viewpoint(11). More recently Bohannan has said:

> The essence of anthropology is simultaneous self-examination and examination of other, unlike peoples. Self-examination is always difficult. Social and cultural self-examination is doubly difficult because social relationships, personalities and ideas are abstract, unlike pots or stone axes. . . . The theme of the discipline is the story of the mastering of human animality by processes and techniques of self-recognition(12).

There is, however, some evidence of an inability to realistically incorporate study and appreciation of psychological phenomenon in the anthropological curriculum. It is not usual for anthropologists to describe their own activities and their responses to the challenges of living in strange environmental and sociocultural settings. In the teaching and utilization of process recordings, the nurse has developed a methodology which permits her to objectify and analyze her own behavior in the clinical context. This is a contribution which nursing can make to anthropological studies.

Although anthropology is the holistic study of man, there is a tendency towards narrow specialization on the part of individual anthropologists. Nurses can assist those anthropologists who maintain interests and study primarily in social anthropology, cultural anthropology, or culture and personality to obtain greater awareness, understanding, and appreciation of the biological dimension of man.

Nurses also participate and exercise some measure of control in a great variety of clinical settings. For the anthropologist the clinical setting is conceptualized as a natural setting in which natural phenomena may be examined. These settings have great potential for much useful and creative anthropological study of benefit to both anthropology and nursing. Collaborations between anthropologists and nurses would facilitate the anthropologist's entree into the clinical setting. In such collaborations nurses can provide professional conceptualizations and descriptions of interpersonal action in the clinical setting which would facilitate problem identification and problem solving.

Issues related to the introduction of new health care programs are particularly compatible with the anthropological study of social and cultural change. Adams has noted the fruitfulness of collaborations between public health programmers and anthropologists(13). Adams believed that the particular contribution of anthropology is the delineation and clarification of cultural and subcultural social systems and belief systems which have an impact upon new health programs. As noted previously, the development of such collaborations usually has a salutary effect upon the more equal distribution of quality health services.

Such collaborations do not require that nurses merely provide the anthropologists with information, clinical (natural) settings, and opportunities for study. Prepared nurses can participate in such studies as "key" informants. As applied scientists they can also participate in problem identification, data gathering, and data analysis. The studies of Seymour Parker and other investigators are suggestive of this type of collaboration(14).

Finally, it should be noted that there is, in anthropology, a long tradition of understanding, appreciation, and acceptance of the contributions of women. Among the ranks of female anthropologists are such important names as Margaret Mead, Ruth Benedict, Helen Codere, Cora Du Bois, Else Clews Parsons, Ruth Underhill, Audrey Richards, Ruth Useem, Hortense Powdermaker, Lucy Mair, and Florence Kluckhohn.

CONCLUSIONS

Increasingly, undergraduate and graduate collegiate nursing students are including anthropology as part of their studies. For this reason, this discussion of the contributions which nursing and anthropology can make to each other would not be complete without noting an important similarity in the approach to training of candidates in these two fields. In a recent discussion of graduate study in the United States, Jenks and Reisman complained of a disparagement of practical experience as acceptable for credits and as criteria for the Ph.D. They did note, however, that:

> In anthropology 'field work' in an alien culture is still regarded as having education value above and beyond the data collected, but few other disciplines have comparable requirements. This has remained true despite the increasing availability of second-hand data, and is a tribute to the anthropologists' awareness that socialization of apprentices depends on what they have done as well as what they have read(15).

To a great extent nursing utilizes the clinical setting as the anthropologist utilizes the field. In addition to the care and treatment of the ill the nursing student and the professional nurse practitioner utilize the clinical setting to gather data which will help them to develop their nursing competencies. As it is with the anthropologist in the field, so it is in the clinical setting that socialization, to the discipline occurs. Unlike the anthropological students' field experience, however, the student nurses' clinical experience is usually a directed experience. That is, her clinical activities are closely related to the objectives of her different courses. Her clinical experiences can also be contrasted with the medical students' clinical apprentice-type training.

In order to illuminate certain aspects of its practice, solve some of its problems and develop its theory, nursing has borrowed from many academic and professional disciplines. Yet, it appears that anthropology, the discipline from which nursing has borrowed the least, has much to offer the profession.

SUMMARY

This paper discusses the many intellectual and methodological similarities which exist between anthropology and nursing. It concludes that in the academic discipline of anthropology there is content, method, and a perspective which can be of value to the nurse

and the developing nursing science. There is, also, much in the objectives, practice, and organization of nursing which can be of value to anthropology.

REFERENCES

1. Jaco, E. G. *Patients, Physicians and Illness.* Glencoe, Ill., Free Press, 1958, pp. 3-8.
2. Matarazzo, J. D. Comprehensive medicine; a new era in medical education. *Hum Org* 14:4-9, Spring 1955.
3. Bohannan, Paul. *Social Anthropology.* New York, Holt, Rinehart and Winston, 1963, p. V.
4. Beals, R. L., and Hoijer, Harry. *Introduction to Anthropology.* 3d ed. New York, Macmillan Co., 1965.
5. Fox, Robin. *Kinship and Marriage.* Baltimore, Md. Penguin Books, 1968, p. 11. (Paperback)
6. Hulse, F. S. *Human Species.* New York, Random House, 1963, pp. 459-462.
7. Barnouw, Victor. *Culture and Personality.* Homewood, Ill., Dorsey Press, 1963, p. 3.
8. Kluckhohn, C. K., and Murray, H. A. Eds. *Personality in Nature, Society, Culture.* rev. ed. New York, Alfred A. Knopf, 1953.
9. Kelly, Cynthia H. Detroit-since last Summer. *Amer J Nurs* 68:1278-1292, June 1968.
10. Bohannan, *op. cit., p. v.*
11. Malinowski, Bronislaw. *Argonauts of the Western Pacific.* Prospect Heights, IL: Waveland Press, Inc., 1961 (reissued 1984), pp. 1-26.
12. Bohannon, *op. cit.*, p. 12.
13. Adams, R. N. On the effective use of anthropology in public health programs. *Hum Org* 13:5-15, Winter 1955.
14. Parker, Seymour. Leadership patterns in a psychiatric ward. *Hum Relat* 11(4):287-301, 1958.
15. Jencks, Christopher, and Riesman, David. Where graduate schools fail. *Atlantic* 221:51, Feb. 1968.

A Model for Applied Anthropology

GEORGE M. FOSTER

Nursing is an applied discipline whose major concern is with the improvement of patient care, and improvement implies change. Nursing, however, is attached to institutions, and institutions do not change without a valid reason. Consequently, nursing must, through research, provide facts to prove that a change will enhance the work of the institution and will be worth the time and trouble inherent in learning a different way of doing things. Since the goal of nursing research, either directly or indirectly, is to improve patient care, nursing research can be termed applied research. Foster has defined applied research as having the goal of improving the human condition; and improved patient care is directly involved with that goal.

Although nurses can and do involve themselves in pure research, nursing practice is based upon clinical research, and clinical research meets the requirements of applied research as defined by Foster. Applied research is action oriented: it changes something, and it evaluates the outcome of that change. Clinical nursing research focuses upon nursing interventions, the action portion of nursing care, and evaluates the outcomes of changed nursing practices. Applied research, of whatever nature, requires basic knowledge about the person who is to be changed (usually in terms of behavioral change), the person who is instituting the change, and finally the situation in which the change is to occur. For nursing, these requirements can be translated into a knowledge about the nurse, the patient, and the health situation in which the nursing process occurs.

Applied transcultural nursing research requires basic knowledge of the patient, the nurse, and the health-care institution from the cultural context in order to bring about improved nursing interventions.

THEORETICAL AND APPLIED SCIENCE

We have already considered examples of human problems in technological change of the kind that have given rise to the subdiscipline of applied anthropology, and summarized cases of the work anthropologists have done in several instances. We did not, however, define "applied anthropology" and "applied anthropologist," nor did we discuss the question of how the work of applied anthropologists differs from that of other anthropologists. In this chapter we will examine the relationship between theoretical and applied anthropology, by showing how the role of applied anthropologist fits into the wider scheme of the application of theoretical science to practical problems. By so doing we will outline the necessary conceptual framework for the following chapters, which deal with research methodology, the subject matter of applied anthropological research, the problems of integration of applied anthropologists into technical aid organizations, and the prestige level of applied anthropology as viewed by anthropologists.

At the risk of great oversimplification, we can say that science has two major aspects: *discovery*, the search for and the finding of new phenomena and new relationships between already known phenomena, which are accounted for by the formulation of hypotheses, principles, and scientific laws; and *utilization*, the application of the fruits of discovery and resulting theory in the service of mankind. The first is called "pure" or "basic" or "theoretical" science, and the second, "applied" science. In the popular mind, utilization flows directly from discovery and theory, so that the two aspects of science appear to form one process in which different kinds of personnel participate.

CHART 1 THE POPULAR CONCEPT OF APPLIED SCIENCE

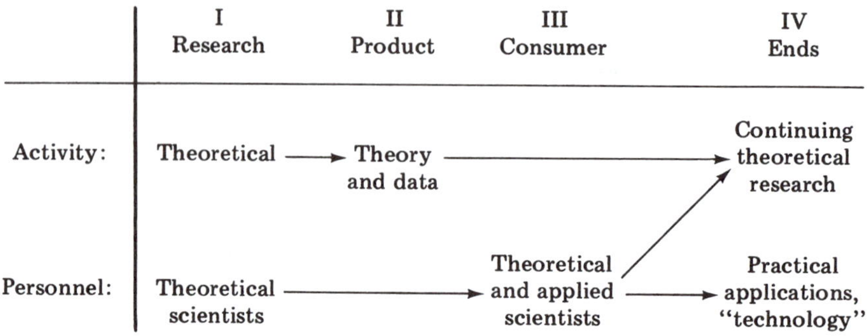

	I Research	II Product	III Consumer	IV Ends
Activity:	Theoretical →	Theory and data →		Continuing theoretical research
Personnel:	Theoretical scientists →		Theoretical and applied scientists → (↗ Continuing theoretical research)	Practical applications, "technology"

Chart 1 illustrates the relationship between pure and applied science as it is popularly conceived, dividing the research-to-use sequence into two elements, the *activity* itself and the *personnel* involved. Theoretical research is seen as carried out by theoretically oriented scientists (Column I), with a resulting "product" of theory and data (Column II). The two kinds of "consumers" of theory and data, theoretical and applied scientists (Column III), each apply the scientific product to their special "ends" (Column IV).

For the theoretically oriented scientist the corpus of scientific data and theory which characterizes his discipline at a given time is merely a progress report, a statement about the condition of the field as it is known up to that time. The product of research, therefore, is merely the jumping-off point for continuing investigation and the search for ever better and more comprehensive theory. For the applied scientist the challenge of knowledge is the search for ways to translate it into forms that will meet the needs of society: consumer goods, medical services, transportation, communication, and recreation and leisure activities. The applied scientist who converts basic knowledge into usable form is commonly thought of as the inventor or the technologist, whose peculiar genius lies in his ability to "work out" ways in which abstract theory can be translated into industrial and other goods and services which make for an ever higher standard of living.

The sequence seems simple: brilliant, theoretical minds produce basic theory, and practical, inventive minds "apply" this theory to the problems of everyday life. Hence we have "applied science." In the exact sciences, in which with some justification we can speak of scientific laws, and in which theory, although stated in problematic terms, permits prediction with certainty, this model of the application of science has a certain validity. Even here, though, it is well to remember that the model is pertinent only in the most general sense, for technology frequently has outrun theory, and in so doing has in fact been a source of that very theory from which it is supposed to draw its sustenance. For example, Pasteur's contributions to bacteriology resulted initially from trying to find solutions to the practical problems of the French silk and wine industries.

THEORETICAL AND APPLIED ANTHROPOLOGY

A great many social scientists, anthropologists among them, have accepted this model uncritically and have assumed that it also fits their disciplines. Many years ago, Radcliffe-Brown wrote that "Applied anthropology must, of course, be based on pure anthropology. What is therefore necessary in the first place is the development of the pure science by the discovery or formulation of the fundamental principles of social integration" (1931:276). Much later Lucy Mair, speaking of the relationships between theoretical and applied science, wrote that "In the field which this discussion generally covers [applied anthropology and development policies] there is no doubt as to what is meant by applied science. It is the application of principles experimentally established to the production of specific results" (1957:9).

Applied anthropology so conceived would simply have to be the application to practical ends of the data and theory of theoretical anthropology, something which could not exist until a vigorous theoretical discipline marked by laws permitting prediciton had come into being. An applied anthropologist would be a technician, the social engineer who did the applying. But, as we will see shortly, the activities that have been labeled "applied anthropology" rarely if ever conform to this simple model. There is, in fact, insufficient high-level anthropological theory on which to base a successful applied branch of the discipline, if the model thought characteristic of the exact sciences must also apply to anthropology. Rather, the many and varied contributions of anthropology to practical problems are based on broad general concepts, such as culture, cultural integration, cultural dynamics, values, social structure, and interpersonal relations, and on a methodology which, like the methodologies of other social sciences, makes its unique contributions to an understanding of human behavior and its underlying motivations.

Usually an anthropologist looks upon the groups he studies in applied assignments as communities and cultures or subcultures basically no different from those he customarily analyzes, amenable to the same research methods and conceptual frameworks he uses in theoretically oriented research. The significant difference between theoretical and applied anthropology lies largely in the distinction Hauser made some years ago for the social sciences in general: ". . . not in the point of view or methods of the investigator, not in the nature of the phenomena under investigation, but rather *in the manner in which the problem is selected, in the auspices of the research and in the immediate, as distinguished from long-run, objectives*" (Hauser 1949:209—emphasis added).

A MODEL

Hence, if the complexities of the relationship between theoretical and applied anthropology are to be appreciated, something more elaborate than the simple model is needed. This is outlined in Chart 2, in which the research-to-use sequence is broken down into the same two elements of activity and personnel portrayed in Chart 1. However, in place of a single sequence, this model shows two, one for "pure" and the other for "applied" science.

Both pure and applied research result in a "product" destined to an "end." The product of the former, ideally at least, is theory—hypotheses and generalizations—about society, culture, and human behavior. That is, the research and the conceptual framework within which it is carried out should produce ideas, insights, and hunches, which, with the data simultaneously acquired, permit theoretical interpretations of social and cultural phenomena, whose "end" is not immediate pertinence to practical programs aimed at making the world a better place in which to live. The product of the latter should be ideas, insights, comprehension, and data which lend themselves to the planning and execution of programs aimed at ameliorating specific social and economic ills, or in bringing about improved practices (as in farming or in health habits) which will benefit individuals and their society. The achievement of rather specific kinds of changes in human behavior is thus the basic "end" of applied anthropology.

Although both sequences are shown as independent, they are actually intimately related (as shown by the diagonal broken arrows), for much research carried out in applied settings has been directly relevant to basic anthropological theory and, conversely, pure research has contributed a great deal to applied problems. In fact from a scientific point of view one of the strongest justifications for applied anthropological research is the contribution it makes to our basic corpus of data and concepts. This model may now be examined more closely.

Research Type. In both pure and applied research (Column I) the scientist is the anthropologist. Since "applied anthropologist" is a role rather than an occupation, the anthropologist will usually be a university teacher who combines teaching with both types of research.

CHART 2 THEORETICAL VS. APPLIED RESEARCH: ANTHROPOLOGY

	I Research Type	II Research Selection	III Research Sponsor	IV Product	V Translator	VI Consumer	VII Ends
Activity:	"Pure"			Theory and data			Continuing research, teaching
Personnel:	Anthropologist	Anthropologist	Foundation		None (Text-writer)?	Anthropologist teachers	
Activity:	"Applied"			Limited theory and practical data			Changes in human behavior
Personnel:	Anthropologist	Innovating organization	Innovating organization		Applied anthropologist, anthropologist consultant	Operational personnel	

The important point is that, whether at the moment engaged in pure or applied research, he will have had only one kind of training and preparation. Consequently he will use the same concepts, methodology, and research methods in an applied assignment as in a theoretical analysis, and he will apply the same scientific canons of accuracy, objectivity, and freedom from value judgments. This statement also holds true for the relatively few career applied anthropologists, for they have had the same training as their academic colleagues. Clearly, the difference between pure and applied anthropology lies neither in research nor in the researchers.

Research Selection and Sponsorship. The difference first appears when we consider who decides upon a research problem (Column II) and who sponsors it (Column III). In pure research the anthropologist usually decides the problem. Selection stems from his personal interest, and his recognition that the time is ripe, or that opportunities are present, to add the next increment of knowledge to a particular theme. Pure research tends to be self-generating; science itself is the dynamic, and the ends of science are determinative.

In applied research the innovating organization charged with solving practical problems usually selects the problem, and the ends of this organization rather than those of science are determinative. The anthropologist, by accepting employment in an enterprise whose primary goals are not scientific, commits himself at least partly to the values and ends of this enterprise.

The sponsors of pure and applied research usually are different. An anthropologist pursuing his own research plans looks for support to an organization whose role in society is defined as furthering knowledge for its own sake, whose continued existence does not depend on an immediate practical "payoff." Sometimes this means research funds from a university itself. More often it is support from a private foundation such as Ford, Wenner-Gren, Carnegie, or the Social Science Research Council. Today the United States government, through the National Science Foundation and the National Institutes of Health, has become the largest supporter of pure anthropological research.

Besides giving money, institutions supporting pure research share other characteristics, the most important of which are that they do not utilize nor make a moral or legal claim on the research results stemming from their support, nor do they normally in any way limit the use of these results by the investigator. The anthropologist usually maintains full control over the data that come from his research, he decides how these data are to be presented to other interested persons, and limitations on their use, if any, are self-imposed, based on his ethical judgments.

By contrast, applied research normally is supported by the innovating bureaucracy, the client organization that sets the problem. It expects to use at least some of the research results in the furtherance of its own ends, to have a moral and legal claim on all results, and to be able to limit their use by the anthropologist who gathered them.

In practice, many sponsors of applied anthropological research operate with an extremely light hand, reserving to the scientist considerable latitude in identifying the critical factors that need investigating, within the broad framework of the practical problem, and allowing him much freedom in presenting his research data to professional colleagues in the form of articles, monographs, and papers read at professional meetings. Their concern is that the anthropologist provide them with sufficient information bearing on their problems to justify his support. Once this goal is achieved, and if there are no security problems, the anthropologist usually is free to utilize his data in whatever scientific way he chooses. A sponsoring organization may, in fact, derive considerable prestige and goodwill by a policy of allowing researchers under contract to act as professionals in presenting data and hypotheses to anthropological colleagues.

The Product of Research. The product of research (Column IV), its form of presentation to others, and its mode of utilization are rather different in pure and applied anthropology. The product of pure research, as has been shown, is science in the form of new data, new hypotheses, new statements of regularities, new laws. Its form of presentation is determined by its major audience of other anthropologists, and scientists in closely related fields. Early and tentative results may be read as scientific papers at professional meetings. Often such papers are rewritten, perhaps in the light of professional criticism, and published as articles in professional journals. Larger bodies of data are subjected to more extensive analysis, to be published in monograph or book form. It is important that the researcher himself is charged with the scientific interpretation of his investigations and their communication to his colleagues.

The product of applied research is perhaps more varied. The results of good applied anthropological investigations include a large theoretical component; this, as the broken arrows in the model indicate, feeds into the product of pure research. But applied research, if it fulfills its aims, must also produce "practical" data and theories in the form of information, ideas, insights, and knowledge that are seen as contributing to the solution of the problems which are the concern of the sponsoring organization. And this "practical" information, the goal of the research as far as the client organization is concerned, usually cannot be communicated in the same fashion as the pure researcher communicates with his colleagues. Rather, much more of it is transferred (in the social sciences, at least), in staff meetings, in organizational conferences, and in informal, often social, settings. Much of the information is also presented in the form of memoranda that can be quickly prepared and inexpensively reproduced in small numbers, to reach the policy makers, administrators, and technicians who presumably can utilize it. To these people, the theoretical component of the research is at best of slight interest.

The Translator and the Consumer. So far, the personnel sequence in both pure and applied anthropological research is essentially the same: anthropologists with the same kind of training (often the same individual), utilizing the same research methodology and following common canons of control and objectivity, examine, observe, analyze, and interpret the meaning of a body of data. They then communicate this knowledge in ways designed to be most easily understood by the audiences for whom it is intended. But here the sequence changes. In pure research the principal "consumers" (Column VI) are the anthropologist himself, his professional colleagues in the social sciences, teachers who, whether or not they engage in similar research, are trained in social science, and the interested reading public. In contrast, the results of applied research are "consumed" by specialists representing other professions and disciplines who view these data simply as one factor among a great many orders of factors they must consider in carrying out their work. These operational personnel, as they are called on the chart, are policy makers and planners, program administrators, and technical specialists in such fields as public health, social welfare, agriculture, community development, and the like.

There is less need in pure than in applied investigation for the role of "translator" (Column V), someone who explains to the consumer the meaning of research results. When the consumer is himself a research scientist he shares a common scientific background with the original investigator, and so needs no help in interpreting new data and theory. The consumer who is not primarily a research specialist—perhaps a college teacher or a layman who wishes to know more about the subject—may find a translator helpful. A translator may be a textbook author, often the research scientist himself, or the science popularizer, a professional writer with the skill necessary to translate the ideas and data found in the monographs and papers with which the scientist communicates with his fellows into forms that require less specialized scientific preparation. So the role of translator exists in pure science, but it is less crucial to achieving major ends than in applied research.

The planners, administrators, and technical specialists who are the consumers of applied anthropological research require that data be presented to them in a form they can relate to the other factors they manipulate in their work. The often esoteric terminology of social scientists must be simplified, and the facts critical to a project must be extracted from the mass of data in which they are imbedded, and presented in a clear, succinct manner that makes obvious their implications for program planning and operations. The role of translator is essential. Not infrequently—almost always in anthropology—this role is filled by the research scientist himself. Particularly if he has been in close touch with operational personnel, and thus knows their problems well, he is the best suited of all possible people to serve as translator. In an informal way he probably has been translating throughout the research project as he meets with and talks to project administrators and technicians.

Consultants also fill the role of translators. In anthropology they are usually university professors who are called in by an action-oriented agency for a day or two, or sometimes longer, to try to relate specific anthropological data or basic theory to some problem on which the action agency is working. Sometimes consultants also do short-term research dealing with these problems.

It is at this point in the model that we can properly speak of "application" and of an "applied anthropologist." It is here that the results of a specific action-oriented research project are related to pertinent general anthropological theory and data, purged of their irrelevancies for the ends of the organization that is sponsoring the research, and presented to operational personnel in ways and in forms that permit maximum utilization. It is a mark of the youth of anthropology that the university-based scientist whose primary interest is theoretical research, but who may also engage in action-oriented research from time to time, is usually this translator who fills the temporary role of applied anthropologist. In other sciences this function has long since been assigned to recognized specialists. In the natural sciences the specialist is the industrial scientist or the industrial engineer, while in genetics he is the animal or plant geneticist. Anthropology is moving toward similar specialization, and the time will come when some anthropologists will find their major interests clustering around this type of activity. Already we are beginning to see this in medical anthropology and educational anthropology.

But for some time, at least, the role of translator, of applied anthropologist, will continue to be played by the general, all-purpose anthropologist.

The responsibility of translator, whether assigned to a full-time specialist or temporarily to a university-based scientist, is by no means passive, a mechanical task of finding simple answers to social problems in technological change, and then explaining what it is all about in words and concepts the layman can understand. It is, or should be, a research role in which a high degree of creativity is exercised, and from which significant contributions to basic theory emerge. Often the anthropologist has access to groups of people he could not study in traditional research, and almost always he can learn about the workings of bureaucracy, through real "participant observation," in a way denied to most anthropologists concerned with more traditional tasks.

When a mutually satisfying personal relationship exists between the anthropologist and the administrator, the former will play a major part in the selection of research projects as well as in determination of research design, although of course ultimate authority lies with the administrator. The wise administrator knows his problems and the kinds of answers he needs to solve them, but he recognizes that the anthropologist knows better than he how to get these answers. The applied anthropologist has the responsibility of familiarizing himself with the administrator's (and the technical specialist's) needs, and then telling him what questions are to be asked (i.e., determining research design) in order to meet these needs. For these, and other reasons to be discussed later, the best applied anthropology occurs when there is a close operating relationship, with mutual respect and trust, between the anthropologist and the personnel of the organization charged with reaching specific goals.

Although it is in the role shown as translator on the model that the activities of the applied anthropologist most commonly cluster, applied anthropologists also sometimes serve as administrators. They are then themselves "consumers" of applied research, their own or that of other anthropologists. This was true of the Papaloapan resettlement scheme described earlier, where anthropologist-administrators planned and directed the work, and of the Vicos project. Anthropologists also served, as we have mentioned, as administrators in the War Relocation Authority camps in World War II, and in the Trust Territory of Micronesia following the war. There is no reason why an anthropologist—or any other scientist —should not make a good administrator. Although to the layman the scientist, apparently isolated by his ivy-covered walls from the real world of action, may appear to be the antithesis of the practical administrator, the fact is that the same thought processes, the same analytical methods, and the same judgments characterize both. Scientists and administrators alike must define their goals, decide what the significant data are, acquire these data, order them, and draw conclusions from them. Only at this point does a basic distinction appear. The scientist's task is done when he draws conclusions, i.e., advances his hypotheses. But the administrator is then faced with the most critical test of all: he must take action, based on what has gone before, and hope that his conclusions further his organization's course toward meeting its goals.

Nevertheless, although anthropologists have served as able administrators, there is general agreement among American and British anthropologists that this is not a desirable role *if* the anthropologist also expects to do research. The anthropologist's primary value in goal-oriented projects is that he can be impartial, a friend of the personnel of the bureaucracy and of the members of the target group. In exercising his obligations he does not have to reveal confidences or take action which may impinge on the freedom of others. The administrator, on the other hand, must exercise authority. People are much less apt to be frank informants if they know that the anthropologist to whom they are revealing information may subsequently change hats and use this information to their detriment (as seen by them, at least). So, although anthropologists sometimes work as administrators, this is not the major focal point of applied anthropological activities.

The Ends of Research. The "ends" (Column VII) of theoretical and applied research are distinct. For the theoretician they are additional research, and probably teaching by the anthropologist himself. Thus, the initiator of the original research, and professional colleagues similarly trained, see the sequence through to its logical end. It is an integrated activity without significant discontinuities, all comfortably within the confines of a rather tight little professional group. Anthropologists maintain control at all stages of the sequence, and they are responsible for the ethical and moral as well as the scientific aspects of this sequence. It is an essentially secure situation for the researcher: he has no outside master, and he is responsible to and judged only by his colleagues.

For the applied anthropologist, the ends of the research sequence are changes in human behavior which further modernization, technological and social development, and higher standards of living. Mexican villagers may adopt new health practices as a consequence of research about traditional beliefs which permits a more efficient government health service, or traditional farmers, following upon similar applied research, may be persuaded to adopt improved cultivation methods. But in contrast to the theoretical sequence, the anthropologist who carries out and interprets the research essentially loses control of the operation at the point where administrators and technical specialists begin to use his material. The responsibility for final action lies in their hands, and not in his. For the anthropologist working in an applied setting this loss of control is sometimes disquieting and unsettling. Since the anthropologist tends to identify more with the people who form the target group than with those in the innovating organization, he is sensitive lest in some way confidences revealed to him in the course of research may, if they reach the ears of others, injure the informants. Or he fears that the results of his research may be carelessly or even dishonestly utilized.

The best way to minimize these dangers, I believe, is for the anthropologist to have a close working relationship with the members of the bureaucracy itself. In this way, through personal friendship and through intimate knowledge of the action programs as they shape up and are executed, he can maintain a degree of informal control which in most instances is sufficient to ensure that anthropology's ethical standards are maintained.

A DEFINITION

The activities and personnel roles involved in theoretical and applied anthropology have been compared and contrasted by means of a model. This model points out how an anthropologist is best thought of as doing applied work when he has some kind of formal tie with an innovating organization oriented toward social, economic, and technological goals involving rather specific kinds of changes in human behavior. When working in such a setting, the anthropologist accepts the organization's right to determine the major research topics, in return for which he receives financial and other support. He also agrees to present his research results and the ideas stemming from them to the personnel of the organization in forms acceptable to planners, administrators, and technical specialists, rather than in the forms customarily used to communicate with members of his own discipline. It is this functional association with a nonacademic organization with goals of the type described, and the role modifications that the association requires, that makes an applied anthropologist.

The anthropologist draws upon his basic professional knowledge, of course, but only rarely can it be said that he is "applying" theory and data developed on the "pure" side of the discipline to practical problems. When his applied assignment involves investigation, he works in essentially the same way as when his interest is primarily theoretical, simultaneously bearing in mind both his own questions about human behavior and those asked by the administrators and technicians in the organization with which he is associated.

Stressing association rather than application, we can say that *"applied anthropology" is the phrase commonly used by anthropologists to describe their professional activities in programs that have as primary goals changes in human behavior believed to ameliorate contemporary social, economic, and technological problems, rather than the development of social and cultural theory.*

It may be argued, with some justification, that this definition should be broadened to include research which is neither selected nor supported by a client organization, but whose product is of immediate or potential use in an action program. Thus, Steubing's analysis of the tension that exist in a high school, briefly summarized later, was not supported by an action-oriented organization. Nevertheless his observations would be extremely useful for a school system examining itself with a view to improving operations. The Institute of Social Anthropology's public health research was, in fact, preceded by a shorter research project selected by anthropologist rather than by public health personnel, and supported by Smithsonian Institution funds. The results of this research were recognized by Institute of Inter-American Affairs personnel as significant to their health programs, and this led to the inclusion of anthropologists on the evaluation team. Because of the use immediately made of this initial research it is properly classed as applied, even though the usual bureaucratic ties did not exist. Few, if any, definitions can be completely comprehensive and precise, fitting all conceivable cases. The one-sentence definition above, however, seems to me to be generally accurate, and at the same time expressive of the basic differences between theoretical and applied work.

REFERENCES

Hauser, Philip M. "Social Science and Social Engineering." *Philosophy of Science*, 16:209-218.

Mair, Lucy P. *Studies in Applied Anthropology.* London School of Economics Monographs on Social Anthropology, No. 16. London University of London, The Athlone Press. 1957.

Radcliffe-Brown, A.R. "Applied Anthropology." Report of the Twentieth Meeting of the Australian and New Zealand Associates for the Advancement of Science. Brisbane, Queenland. 1931, pp. 267-280.

Problems and Issues

Nursing, more than any other health profession, is an integrative discipline. Nursing blends, borrows, adapts, and uses knowledge from many fields. Whatever influences patient care is appropriate and necessary. If nursing has a unique body of knowledge, this uniqueness comes from the synthesis of a wide variety of areas of dissimilar content. For nursing, however, content without application is irrelevant. Every aspect of nursing eventually hinges upon the nursing process, and the study of nursing requires analysis of both process and content.

The problems and issues confronting transcultural nursing involve the determination of what aspects of anthropology are most useful to the practice of nursing. Since anthropology defines itself as the study of man, it is as difficult to delineate the parameters of anthropology as of nursing. Each of the four major areas of anthropology (social and cultural anthropology, physical anthropology, linguistics, and archaeology) can contribute to nursing knowledge (with the possible exception of archaeology), and with the development of subfields of anthropology, many more specialties are becoming available to nursing practice. With the exception of the article by Kasselman, the papers in this book focus on the blend of cultural anthropology with nursing.

Cultural anthropology is, itself, an extremely broad and wide-ranging field of study. It encompasses what man believes about life, about himself, about the world around him, and about what he has created; and how man interprets human interaction in terms of symbolism and shared meanings. Man is, basically, a symbolic interactionist. Man interacts with other men in terms of symbols. Social systems, social roles, and language are all symbolic interactions. Man interacts on the basis of rules—rules for behavior, rules for relationships, and rules for knowledge. Rules symbolize organization; they economize interactions through predictability.

Transcultural nursing is also concerned with symbolic interaction: the communication system used by the nurse and the patient; the values and beliefs which guide behavior; the level at which shared meaning occurs; and finally, what happens when cultural barriers are crossed. Nurse and patient interact around the concepts of health and illness. The degree to which they agree on what is health, illness, treatment, and cure will affect their subsequent interactions. When nurse and patient do not share a common language, they are unable to discover whether they agree or not. When they share the same language, but do not agree on the meanings for certain words, their communication will suffer. It is the nurse's responsibility to discover the degree to which the nurse and the patient share the same goals and the same symbols.

The focus of transcultural nursing is health care delivery to the consumer within his cultural context; this requires of the nurse a sensitivity to the differences between her own and the patient's cultural background. The realization that not all people agree with the tenets of the Western system of health care, that not all people espouse the "germ theory," that not all people seek out physicians when they are ill, places the nurse in the position of having to reevaluate her own belief systems and her own health care practices as not always being "the right way" or "the only way" to intervene in illness situations. Many nurses become frustrated with the patient who does not comply with his medical regime, regardless of whether the patient believes in the treatment plan. The process of discovering why the patient has come to be in our Western system of health care, rather than in another, or even if he is using two systems of health care at the same time, is not only revealing but very exciting.

The uncooperative patient, as Frances MacGregor points out, may be a product of a totally different culture. The discovery of the cause of conflict between patients and nurses, and the acceptance by nurses of the patient's beliefs, led to nursing interventions that helped the patients to comply with the medical regimen. Nurses and patients made adjustments, and behavior change occurred in both. Transcultural nursing requires the assessment of both parties in the interaction, since both come to the situation with preconceived notions about the way they should act and the way the other person should respond. The conflicts that arise when expectations are not met become insoluble unless one of the parties makes the attempt to intervene. In the situations described by MacGregor, the responsibility fell to the nurse.

A major area of conflict in a transcultural situation is that of the communication systems used, as Hall and Whyte so clearly describe. When neither the patient nor the nurse make any attempt to understand one another, or worse, have no idea that they are not communicating with one another, the breach between the two becomes wider. The degree to which the nurse realizes that the communication barrier goes beyond that of differing languages, the greater is her potential for crossing that barrier. Although Hall and Whyte speak primarily of different verbal and nonverbal communication systems across cultures, transcultural nursing includes intracultural communication systems within subcultures of the United States. Regional variation, minority languages, and in-group terminologies all form part of transcultural communication, to which the nurse must become sensitive.

What a person believes is reflected in what he says and does, so that mentally tuning in to what a person is saying frequently provides clues to what he values in life. One paradigm for establishing values is offered by Florence Kluckhohn in her paper "Dominant and Variant Value Orientations." This model provides the transcultural nurse with a relatively simple formula for establishing similarities between herself and her client. If the nurse is "future oriented" in her health teaching or in her rehabilitation programs, she will run into difficulties with patients who are "present oriented" toward health and illness. While the nurse is planning for the future, the patient is focusing upon present problems and is not listening. Or, if the nurse believes that every patient should make his own decisions or should be individualistic about his health care, how does she respond to the patient who insists upon going home to discuss the recommendations with his grandfather or in a family conclave. In this situation the nurse expects an immediate decision while the patient feels bound to delay the decision until he has consulted with appropriate relatives. Neither the patient nor the nurse can understand the other's point of view. Or again, the Western trained nurse believes that modern medicine can control or at least combat most of today's diseases, or maintains the hope that in the near future research will produce a "cure" for the particular illness. The client on the other hand is firmly convinced that illness is caused by being "out of balance" with nature or is " the will of God." These value systems are in conflict with one another in the Western system of health care, necessitating an unbiased assessment on the part of the nurse, and a change in her approach to intervention. When the beliefs and values of the patient and nurse coincide, the treatment is enhanced—but when they are in direct conflict, the nurse must assume the responsibility for adapting her behavior to that of the patient.

Interestingly enough, the conflicts that arise in the transcultural setting are not due solely to interpersonal conflicts, but stem from conflicts that arise out of the process of socialization. Each of us has been raised in a particular culture with particular beliefs and values that were handed down to us from our parents, teachers, and peers. As we grow older we are expected to change our behavior to suit our new roles, yet we are not always trained for those roles. With each new role we acquire, whether through aging, education, jobs, marriage, or whatever, we learn to adjust to that role and develop the position to suit ourselves, and in many ways, change the role for the next generation. Because we are not trained for roles, we become enmeshed in change, create change, and transform the culture in which we were raised. Yet the process of being and becoming change agents can be a difficult one, as Ruth Benedict clearly points out.

As nurses, we have experienced the continuities and discontinuities of cultural conditioning in our own nursing education. We are socialized into the role of student nurses, only to become self-sufficient, responsible Registered Nurses on the day we receive our state board results. We become expert clinicians, only to be promoted to administration. The role-strain and feelings of unpreparedness are not so different from the role-strains we experienced as successful children who were forced into adulthood. Despite the awkwardness we feel, we can capitalize upon a seeming failure in preparation by becoming more creative in the new role than we would have been had we been trained for it.

If we can view the discontinuities in cultural conditioning in a positive rather than a negative light, we can view the model presented by Kluckhohn and Mowrer as a means for creating change in a system. Note the idiosyncratic level of personality development. Here we find the individual "accidents" that occur to each of us from the moment of birth. Individual changes must occur before role changes can occur. Role changes lead to social or group change and finally the cultural or universal level may be affected. At present, transcultural nursing occurs on the idiosyncratic level—on an interpersonal accidental basis. However, as more nurses become aware of cultural influences, the development of the role of transcultural nursing will not be far behind.

Again following Kluckhohn and Mowrer's paradigm, nurse-patient interactions within a cultural context can be viewed in relation to the assessment process. What individual biological, sociological, environmental, and cultural accidents are part of the patient's past history that may affect his health care? What of the roles—biological, environmental, social, and cultural—that the client has assumed? What group or universal determinants influence his health behavior? The model adds to the nursing assessment of transcultural variables.

The last issue to be dealt with in this section is that of culture shock, a phenomenon that occurs for both nurses and patients. Not only do nurses care for patients who may be in some phase of culture shock, but nurses who choose to work in other countries may experience this "disease" for themselves. The knowledge that the "shock" may occur in a variety of contexts should be a relief to both nurses and patients who may not be aware of what is happening to them. The utility of such a concept to nursing exemplifies Osborne's contention that the blend of anthropology and nursing has much to offer.

As the literature in medical anthropology grows, and with it transcultural nursing, problems and issues will become clearer. Transcultural diagnostic procedures and treatment modalities will become better known. Research should provide more data on the patient who chooses more than one system of health care, and is successfully able to adapt to both. The Western system of health care may have to develop, eventually, a middleman system between the professional and the client from another culture in order to insure clear communication between the two. As each issue is raised, nurses will take part in the decision making, serving as the advocate for the patient to insure his care within his cultural context.

RECOMMENDED READINGS

Foster, George M., *Applied Anthropology.* Boston: Little, Brown, and Company, 1969.

Hall, Edward T., *The Silent Language.* Greenwich, Conn.: Fawcett Publications, Inc., 1959.

Jaco, Gartly, ed., *Patients, Physicians, and Illness: Sourcebook in Behavioral Science and Medicine.* New York: The Free Press, 1972.

Kluckhohn, Florence Rockwood, and Fred L. Strodbeck, *Variations in Value Orientations.* Elmsford, N.Y.: Row, Peterson and Company, 1961.

Mead, Margaret, "Nursing—Primitive or Civilized," *American Journal of Nursing* 56 (1956):1001-4.

Uncooperative Patients: Some Cultural Interpretations

FRANCES C. MACGREGOR

The issue raised in this very seminal article is that not all patient behaviors can be interpreted through the standard nursing assessment of biological, psychological, and social variables. Misunderstanding can and does occur when the cultural variable is not included as part of nursing assessment. As MacGregor clearly states, the cultural variable exists just as much for the patient who comes from a different region of the country as it does for the foreign patient. Although this article focuses upon the hospitalized patient who has been termed uncooperative by nursing staff, other negative patient labels may have a cultural base as well. The deviant patient, the noncompliant patient, the hostile or belligerent patient, and the malingering patient are all terms which may be viewed from the cultural variable for a possible explanation.

Perhaps one of the most frustrating experiences in nursing is being unable to get patients to do what one wants them to do even when it is for their own good. What appears to be a patient's outright resistance to the medical and nursing regimen designed solely for his well-being and, hopefully, for his recovery can generate in a nurse any number of negative reactions: a sense of failure, helplessness, irritation, or even anger. However rigorously she may have disciplined herself not to reveal emotional responses of this nature, they are usually communicated to her patient in one or several of the ways in which people unconsciously transmit messages.[1] Such messages, more meaningful to patients than is generally recognized, do not ameliorate the situation; rather, they tend to evoke such counter responses as anxiety, withdrawal, or alienation. The resulting impairment of the therapeutic process is often compounded by negative assessments of the noncompliant patient. He is labeled "uncooperative," "difficult," "stubborn," "perverse," or "a problem." Once this occurs, the kind of relationship between nurse and patient which is so important to the latter's welfare and to the former's satisfaction is broken.

When, despite careful explanations and appeals to reason, a patient persistently refuses to take his medication or exercises, for example, or to stay in bed or keep to his diet, several methods are commonly used to alter his behavior. He may be scolded, given less attention, or even threatened with the withdrawal of privileges. Conferences may be held on how to "handle" him, or how to motivate him, or whether to arrange for psychiatric consultation. Sometimes these methods work, but the frequency with which they don't—and especially *why* they don't—should concern anyone interested in improving the quality of patient care.

The behavior of noncompliant patients, however deviant or seemingly inappropriate, is not a matter of mere capriciousness. There are reasons why they respond as they do, and, apart from reasons that are solely physiologic or organic, explanations may be found on other levels: psychologic, sociologic, and/or cultural. This paper will deal with behavior that is culturally conditioned.

The customs of a group of people, learned, shared, and transmitted from one generation to another are known as their culture. In each culture there is a characteristic way of life within which the individual acquires a language, food habits, religious practices, a style of dress, and so on. These, as well as such subtle things as the way he responds to pain, his reactions toward fear, and his attitudes toward modesty, distinquish him from members of another culture.

[1] For example, on a paralinguistic level (tone of voice), kinesic level (expressive behavior of the body), proxemic level (spatial behavior), or tacticle level (touch).

One cannot underestimate the tenacity of cultural patterns and the hold they have on patients even when health is at stake. Such things as ethnic and social class background and religion are all sources of differential responses to illness and treatment, and the violation of health requirements by many patients stems from these differentials. Unless a nurse learns to think in cultural terms, just as she learns to think in psychologic terms, she will continue to be baffled, if not exasperated, on such occasions.

A recent case in point was that of Mr. G., aged 30, hospitalized with coronary artery disease. Complete quiet and bed rest were prescribed. Several hours after admission, a nurse was shocked to find him out of bed, standing and gazing out of the window. He was promptly helped back to bed and admonished for this infraction of orders. The next day, not once but several times, he was discovered standing by the window. What was the matter with this patient? the nurses asked. Did he not comprehend the seriousness of his condition? Did he lack common sense or was he self-destructive? No one had thought to ask him why he deliberately disobeyed orders, and in view of his behavior he was considered a "real problem."

The explanation for Mr. G.'s persistence in ignoring the rules was not hard to find, though it could well have been overlooked. A nurse who did think in terms of people's cultural backgrounds pointed out that he came from India, a fact that might be related to his actions. A subsequent talk with him revealed that, as a Moslem believer, he was obliged to look toward Mecca to pray, five times a day. For him, religious practices took priority over doctors' orders and considerations of health. The solution was simple: Mr. G.'s bed was moved to a position from which he could face the prescribed direction for worship.

Misunderstandings often have their roots in cross-cultural communication and in the differences in expectations of the persons involved. I am not referring here to communication problems that stem from language differences, but to those problems that arise when, because a common language is spoken, we assume we understand, but we don't. Mr. B., for example, a Swedish patient who spoke fluent English, had become something of a puzzle to the nursing staff. Since his surgery he had invariably responded by "no, thank you" to their offers of water, fruit juice, and back rubs, all of which would have aided his comfort and ultimate recovery. The nurses were even more perplexed (and indignant as well) when his wife complained about his nursing care on the basis of his report that he was not receiving these attentions. Hearing the nurses vent their feelings about Mr. and Mrs. B., a nursing student of Swedish origin volunteered the information that, when proffering food or other attentions,

Swedes customarily repeat the offer two or three times. In turn, to avoid appearing overly eager, Swedish etiquette requires the intended recipient to decline the offer until pressed to accept.

Here indeed was the reasons for the impasse with Mr. B. While he and the nurses spoke the same language, the difference in cultural expectations had led to misinterpretation. Neither the patient nor the staff had realized that each was conveying a message which the spoken words did not make explicit.

Americans pride themselves on being direct and to the point. A response of "no, thank you" is generally taken at face value. Social etiquette is not necessarily breached by failure to insist on acceptance. On the contrary, repeated urging tends to be viewed as poor form. Mr. B., however, though he wanted attention, was following the ritualistic device prescribed by his culture; he felt slighted when the nurses did not repeat their offers.

Though explanations for many events similar to the one just described depends as did these on small understandings, the cultural components that operate in other situations are not always so easily and fortuitously uncovered. As in the following situation, the sources of behavior may be more elusive and complex.

Mrs. R., aged 68, had had both legs amputated as a result of peripheral vascular disease. Since nicotine causes constriction of the peripheral blood vessels., Mrs. R., a heavy smoker, had been told she must stop smoking. It quickly became clear, however, that she was not cooperating. To prevent progression of the disease in the upper extremities and further circulatory complications that might even lead to death, the nursing staff set for themselves an apparently simple goal: to keep Mrs. R. from smoking. Assuming that she understood and accepted their explanation about why she should not smoke, the two nursing students assigned to care for her tried to help by removing her cigarettes and keeping an eye out for hidden ones. Mrs. R. thereupon accused them of "punishing" her and of acting like "bosses" or like "depriving mothers." Similarly, other therapeutic procedures that she disliked, such as heat lamp treatments or being removed from her wheelchair, she saw as "punishment" and being "ordered around." When the students attempted to convince her that what they were doing, particularly the confiscation of cigarettes, was not punishment but necessary to avoid future complications, she would pat their faces and say: "Yes, yes, I know—but I'm not really a big smoker." And before long she was smoking again.

Repeated explanations, scoldings, and even threats of dire consequences were of no avail. The students, who were both concerned and challenged by Mrs. R.'s attitude toward restrictions designed for her benefit, asked themselves an appropriate question: What meaning does smoking have for her? If, they argued, we can find out what lies behind her disregard of the doctor's orders, perhaps we can win her cooperation and solve this problem.

They turned to their instructors for possible explanations. One instructor suggested that Mrs. R. was unable to give up smoking because she was addicted to nicotine. A psychiatric nurse advanced the theory that smoking for this particular patient was a means of satisfying dependency needs. They noted that her unconscious orientation to life appeared to be an oral one, as evidenced by her talkativeness and frequent nibbling on fruit between meals, not because of hunger but probably to satisfy deeper needs. Smoking was simply another means of oral gratification. The students were reminded also that Mrs. R.'s resistance to other forms of therapy was no doubt a "manifestation of hostility on a passible level." It was observed that since she had been warned of the serious consequences of smoking, her deliberate continuance was in actuality a "suicidal ideation." Though the students gave careful consideration to these theories and interpretations, they were able neither to substantiate them nor to put them to immediate use. Mrs. R. continued to smoke.

The students' next avenue of exploration was Mrs. R.'s background. She had been born in Czechoslovakia and had come to the United States when she was 15 years old. At age 22 she married a native-born Czech. She had had the equivalent of a high school education. For many years (until the onset of illness) she had worked as a maid in a college dormitory. She spoke fluent English, but in the Czech community where she lived she continued to speak her native tongue. Although she had been in the United States for more than 50 years, her acculturation was for the most part superficial.

The students next turned their attention to an examination of the cultural characteristics of Czechs as acquired through child-rearing practices. According to Wolfenstein, a distinctive disciplinary technique of Czech mothers is that of combining reward and punishment (1). For example, the child is promised long in advance that if he is good he will receive a reward.

Meanwhile, if the child should misbehave, he is threatened with the withholding of this promised treat. On their part, the children tend to react to what they feel are unfair demands or deprivations by behavior that is just the opposite of what the mother wants. For example, a mother put her child in the corner for being naughty. Told later that she could come out, the child replied: "Thank you, now I like it here"(2). Wolfenstein has hypothesized that such perversity serves both to disappoint the mother and to show her that the child will not be bossed(2).

The tendency of Czechs to resist orders and to react by opposites to authority, their strong dislike of supervision or domination, and their insistence upon autonomy have been noted by students of Czech culture and by Czechs themselves. Even the Czech's concept of his body is one of autonomy: "It is mine to do with as I like, even if it means self-destruction." To demand cooperation from the Czech, then, seems likely to meet with failure, because of method of training.

When he is ill, the adult Czech is no different from many other patients in his tendency to regress to a childlike state. Early behavior patterns become reactivated, and he feels like and often acts like a child. His behavior is determined in large part by the family and the cultural milieu in which he has been reared. The sick adult also, as studies have shown, tend to regard the doctor and nurse as father and mother: authority figures who can both punish and reward. Again, the patient interprets their ministrations and reacts to them in the light of his past experience.

Following the clues provided by their investigation of Czech patterns of behavior, the students hypothesized that Mrs. R.'s withholding of cooperation might be a cultural response to what she perceived as punishment and unfair deprivation, and as being "bossed." If this were true, it could explain their failure to obtain her cooperation in the therapeutic regimen. A shift of tactics seemed indicated. The students stopped scolding and threatening. They deliberately left cigarettes on Mrs. R.'s bedside table, explaining that the decision about smoking was her own to make. In the week that followed there were marked changes. Mrs. R.'s smoking was substantially cut down, and her resistance to nursing procedures lessened as well. For the first time she was receptive to treatment and became actively interested in plans for future therapy and home care.

Obviously, we cannot conclude that cultural components alone were operating in this patient's behavior. Moreover, it would be difficult to separate out each and all of the factors that possibly played a role or to determine the extent to which each operated. Whether or not she was motivated in part by what psychiatrists call "oral careful assessment of the patient, as would the assumption about her "hostility." From the information we do have, however, the cultural components appear to be dominant in this patient's response to treatment.

By presenting this case in some detail the intent has been to demonstrate: (1) the degree to which early cultural conditioning governs people's attitudes and reactions, (2) the importance of viewing a patient within the context of his cultural orientation rather than as an individual in a social vacuum, and (3) how knowledge of a patient's cultural heritage can provide insights that may lead to better management and prevent self-destructive consequences.

One may well wonder how a nurse can be a walking encyclopedia on the ethnic and social background represented by her patients. Obviously, she cannot. Even though research is constantly adding to our knowledge of cultural characteristics of different peoples, there is no compendium she can use for a quick check.

What, then, can the nurse do when she has patients who are uncooperative or whose responses to treatment interfere with specific nursing goals? If she is aware of the meaning of culture, she will know that many of her patients' attitudes and reactions, "strange" or "different" as they seem to her, reflect particular cultures, just as her attitudes and reactions in large measure reflect hers. Instead of making moralistic judgments or ascribing the behavior to some personality idiosyncrasy, she will ask: Is there something about the fact that this patient is a Czech, an Italian, a Mexican, a Jew, a Chinese, or a Frenchman that may have relevance for his behavior? Moreover, she will not limit this question to recently arrived nationals, nor to those who may be second-generation Americans. She will ask the same question if the patient happens to come from another region of the United States such as the Deep South, New England, or the Southwest, or even from a social class different from hers. For here also one finds contrasts in behavior that are the reflection of subcultural backgrounds. These are as important as are the more conspicuous racial and ethnic differences.

By considering alternative possibilities for patients' behaviors, the dangers inherent in making interpretations from a single frame of reference or from one disciplinary approach will be avoided. For example, there is a tendency for medical and nursing personnel to explain difficulties in terms of personality characteristics, and to seek in depth psychology or in Freudian psychiatry explanations for behavior they regard as deviant, resistive, or inappropriate. Emphasis is given to psychologic determinants, and a patient is said to be "hostile," "neurotic," "aggressive," or "acting out." Yet it is not uncommon to discover—and usually to the patient's disadvantage—that a psychologic interpretation has masked what is actually a cultural problem, and that his behavior seen in the larger sociocultural matrix is quite appropriate.

In my work with both nursing staff and students I have found that once cultural awareness has developed, the uncooperative patient is more likely to be perceived as a challenge than a problem. Such awareness does not require the expertise of a cultural anthropologist.

What it does require is recognition of differences in patients; in their value orientations; and in their attitudes toward illness, hospitalization, and treatment, coupled with a readiness to make allowances for them.

Such sensitivity fosters mutual benefits: more effective care for patients, and less frustration for nurses.

REFERENCES

1. Wolfenstein, Martha. Some variants in moral training of children. In *Childhood in Contemporary Cultures*, edited by Margaret Mead and Martha Wolfenstein. 1st ed. Chicago, Ill., University of Chicago Press, 1955, chapter 21, pp. 349-368.
2. *Ibid.*, p. 361.

Intercultural Communication: A Guide to Men of Action

EDWARD T. HALL / WILLIAM FOOTE WHYTE

Nurse-patient interactions always occur within a communication context (whether verbal or nonverbal), and nursing assessment is based upon that interaction. Communication is a series of symbols designating the meanings of things or events that have been learned within a cultural context. Language is a shared system of symbols which can be taught and understood by the members of the in-group. Language is immediately obvious to the listener and speaker—they agree that the language is familiar or unintelligible. Nonverbal communication is not so easy to define. Each person believes that his system of sign language is universally known and understood and each expects the other to understand.

Hall and Whyte direct our attention to the confusion and misunderstandings that arise in intercultural communication when each party expects the other to understand his meaning. The article is easily translated into nurse-patient interactions. When the nurse and the patient agree that they do not share the same language, an interpreter can be found, and should be found immediately. But nurses use medical terms that are frequently unintelligible to English speakers, or expect patients to understand the purposes for some of the gadgetry in hospital settings. The use of colloquial expressions to indicate bodily functions may not be shared. Understanding the

Reproduced by permission of the Society for Applied Anthropology from *Human Organization*, 19, No. 1 (1960):5-12.

principles of intercultural communication assists the nurse in her assessment process.

How can anthropological knowledge help the man of action in dealing with people of another culture? We shall seek to answer that question by examining the process of intercultural communication.

Anthropologists have long claimed that a knowledge of culture is valuable to the administrator. More and more people in business and government are willing to take this claim seriously, but they ask that we put culture to them in terms they can understand and act upon.

When the layman thinks of culture, he is likely to think in terms of 1) the way people dress, 2) the beliefs they hold, and 3) the customs they practice—with an accent upon the esoteric. Without undertaking any comprehensive definition, we can concede that all three are aspects of culture, and yet point out that they do not get us very far, either theoretically or practically.

Dress is misleading, if we assume that differences in dress indicate differences in belief and behavior. If that were the case, then we should expect to find people dressed like ourselves to be thinking and acting like ourselves. While there are still peoples wearing "colorful" apparel quite different from ours, we find in many industrializing societies that the people with whom we deal dress much as we do—and yet think and act quite differently.

Knowledge of beliefs may leave us up in the air because the connections between beliefs and behavior are seldom obvious. In the case of religious beliefs, we may know, for example, that the Mohammedan must pray to Allah a certain number of times a day and that therefore the working day must provide for praying time. This is important, to be sure, but the point is so obvious that it is unlikely to be overlooked by anyone. The administrator must also grasp the less dramatic aspects of everyday behavior, and here a knowledge of beliefs is a very imperfect guide.

Customs provide more guidance, providing we do not limit ourselves to the esoteric and also search for the pattern of behavior into which a given custom fits. The anthropologist, in dealing with customary behavior, is not content with identifying individual items. To him, these items are not miscellaneous. They have meaning only as they are fitted together into a pattern.

But even assuming that the pattern can be communicated to the administrator, there is still something important lacking. The pattern show how the people act—when among themselves. The administrator is not directly concerned with that situation. Whatever background information he has, he needs to interpret to himself how the people act *in relation to himself*. He is dealing with a cross-cultural situation. The link between the two cultures is provided by acts of communication between the administrator, representing one culture, and people representing another. If communication is effective, then understanding grows with collaborative action. If communication is faulty, then no book knowledge or culture can assure effective action.

This is not to devalue the knowledge of culture that can be provided by the anthropologist. It is only to suggest that the point of implementation of the knowledge must be in the communication process. Let us therefore examine the process of intercultural communication. By so doing we can accomplish two things:

A. Broaden knowledge of ourselves by revealing some of our own unconscious communicative acts.
B. Clear away heretofore almost insurmountable obstacles to understanding in the cross-cultural process.

We also learn that communication, as it is used here, goes far beyond words and includes many other acts upon which judgments are based of what is transpiring and from which we draw conclusions as to what has occurred in the past.

Culture affects communication in various ways. It determines the time and timing of interpersonal events, the places where it is appropriate to discuss particular topics, the physical distance separating one speaker from another, the tone of voice that is appropriate to the subject matter. Culture, in this sense, delineates the amount and type of physical contact, if any, which convention permits or demands, and the intensity of emotion which goes with it. Culture includes the relationship of *what is said to what is meant*—as when "no" means "maybe" and "tomorrow" means "never." Culture, too, determines whether a given matter—say, a business contract—should be initially discussed between two persons or backed out in a day-long conference which includes four or five senior officials from each side, with perhaps an assist from the little man who brings in the coffee.

These are important matters which the businessman who hopes to trade abroad ignores at his peril. They are also elusive, for every man takes his own culture for granted. Even a well-informed national of another country is hard put to explain why, in his own land, the custom is thus-and-so rather than so-and-thus; as hard put, indeed, as you would probably be if asked what is the "rule" which governs the precise time in a relationship that you begin using another man's first name. One "just knows." In other words, you do not know and cannot explain satisfactorily because you learn this sort of thing unconsciously in your upbringing, in your culture, and you take such knowledge for granted. Yet the impact of culture on communication can be observed and the lessons taught.

Since the most obvious form of communication is by language, we will first consider words, meanings, voice tones, emotions, and physical contact; then take up, in turn, the cultural impact of time, place, and social class relations on business situations in various lands. Finally, we will suggest what the individual administrator may do to increase his effectiveness abroad, and what students of culture may do to advance this application of anthropology.

BEYOND LANGUAGE

Americans are often accused of not being very good at language, or at least not very much interested in learning foreign languages. There is little evidence that any people are inherently "better" at languages than any other, given the opportunity and incentive to learn. The West and Central European who has since childhood been in daily contact with two or three languages learns to speak them all, and frequently to read and write them as well. Under similar conditions, American children do the same. Indeed, a not uncommon sight on the backroads of Western Europe is a mute, red-faced American military family lost on a Sunday drive while the youngest child, barely able to lisp his own English, leans from the window to interpret the directions of some gnarled farmer whose dialect is largely unintelligible to most of his own countrymen.

We should not underestimate the damage our lack of language facility as a nation has done to our relations all over the world. Obviously, if you cannot speak a man's language, you are terribly handicapped in communicating with him.

But languages can be learned and yet most, if not all, of the disabling errors described in this article could still be made. Vocabulary, grammar, even verbal facility are not enough. Unless a man understands the subtle cues that are implicit in language, tone, gestures and expression, he will not only consistently misinterpret what is said to him, but he may offend irretrievably without knowing how or why.

DO THEY MEAN WHAT THEY SAY?

Can't you believe what a man says? We all recognize that the basic honesty of the speaker is involved. What we often fail to recognize, however, is that the question involves cultural influences that have nothing to do with the honesty or dependability of the individual.

In the United States we put a premium on direct expression. The "good" American is supposed to say what he means and to mean what he says. If, on important matters, we discover that someone spoke deviously or evasively, we would be inclined to regard him thereafter as unreliable if not out-and-out dishonest.

In some other cultures, the words and their meanings do not have such a direct connection. People may be more concerned with the emotional context of the situation than with the meaning of particular words. This leads them to give an agreeable and pleasant answer to a question when a literal, factual answer might be unpleasant or embarrassing.

This situation is not unknown in our culture, of course. How many times have you muttered your delighted appreciation for a boring evening? We term this simple politeness and understand each other perfectly.

On the other hand, analogous "polite" behavior on a matter of factory production would be incomprehensible. An American businessman would be most unlikely to question another businessman's word if he were technically qualified and said that his plant could produce 1000 gross of widgets a month. We are "taught" that it is none of our business to inquire too deeply into the details of his production system. This would be prying and might be considered an attempt to steal his operational plans.

Yet this cultural pattern has trapped many an American into believing that when a Japanese manufacturer answered a direct question with the reply that he could produce 1000 gross of widgets, he meant what he said. If the American had been escorted through the factory and saw quite clearly that its capacity was, at the most, perhaps 500 gross of widgets per month, he would be likely to say to himself:

> Well, this fellow probably has a brother-in-law who has a factory who can make up the difference. He isn't telling the whole story because he's afraid I might try to make a better deal with the brother-in-law. Besides, what business is it of mine, so long as he meets the schedule?

The cables begin to burn after the American returns home and only 500 gross of widgets arrive each month.

What the American did not know was that in Japanese culture one avoids the direct question unless the questioner is absolutely certain that the answer will not embarrass the Japanese businessman in any way whatsoever. In Japan for one to admit being unable to perform a given operation or measure up to a given standard means a bitter loss of face. Given a foreigner who is so stupid, ignorant, or insensitive as to ask an embarrassing question, the Japanese is likely to choose what appears to him the lesser of two evils.

Americans caught in this cross-cultural communications trap are apt to feel doubly deceived because the Japanese manufacturer may well be an established and respected member of the business community.

EXCITABLE PEOPLE?

Man communicates not by words alone. His tone of voice, his facial expressions, his gestures all contribute to the infinitely varied calculus of meaning. But the confusion of tongues is more than matched by the confusion of gesture and other culture cues. One man's nod is another man's negative. Each culture has its own rich array of meaningful signs, symbols, gestures, emotional connotations, historical references, traditional responses and—equally significant—pointed silences. These have been built up over the millennia as (who can say?) snarls, growls, and love murmurs gathered meaning and dignity with long use, to end up perhaps as the worn coinage of trite expression.

Consider the Anglo-Saxon tradition of preserving one's calm. The American is taught by his culture to suppress his feelings. He is conditioned to regard emotion as generally bad (except in weak women who can't help themselves) and a stern self-control as good. The more important a matter, the more solemn and outwardly dispassionate he is likely to be. A cool head, granite visage, dispassionate logic—it is no accident that the Western story hero consistently displays these characteristics.

In the Middle East it is otherwise. From childhood, the Arab is permitted, even encouraged, to express his feelings without inhibition. Grown men can weep, shout, gesture expressively and violently, jump up and down—and be admired as sincere.

The modulated, controlled Anglo-Saxon is likely to be regarded with suspicion—he must be hiding something, practicing to deceive.

The exuberant and emotional Arab is likely to disturb the Anglo-Saxon, cause him to writhe inwardly with embarrassment—for isn't this childish behavior? And aren't things getting rather out of hand?

Then, again, there is the matter of how loudly one should talk.

In the Arab world, in discussions among equals, the men attain a decibel level that would be considered aggressive, objectionable, and obnoxious in the United States. Loudness connotes strength and sincerity among Arabs; a soft tone implies weakness, deviousness.

This is so "right" in the Arab culture that several Arabs have told us they discounted anything heard over the "Voice of America" because the signal was so weak!

Personal status modulates voice tone, however, even in Arab society. The Saudi Arab shows respect to his superior—to a sheik, say—by lowering his voice and mumbling. The affluent American may also be addressed in this fashion, making almost impossible an already difficult situation. Since in the American culture one unconsciously "asks" another to raise his voice by raising one's own, the American speaks louder. This lowers the Arab's tone more and increases the mumble. This triggers a shouting response in the American—which cues the Arab into a frightened "I'm not being respectful enough" tone well below audibility.

They are not likely to part with much respect for each other.

TO TOUCH OR NOT TO TOUCH?

How much physical contact should appropriately accompany social or business conversation?

In the United States we discourage physical contact, particularly between adult males. The most common physical contact is the handshake and, compared to Europeans, we use it sparingly.

The handshake is the most detached and impersonal form of greeting or farewell in Latin America. Somewhat more friendly is the left hand placed on another man's shoulder during a handshake. Definitely more intimate and warm is the "*doble abrazo*" in which two men embrace by placing their arms around each other's shoulders.

These are not difficult conventions to live with, particularly since the North American can easily permit the Latin American to take the initiative in any form of contact more intimate than the handshake. Far more difficult for the North American to learn to live with comfortably are the less stylized forms of physical contact such as the hand on one's arm during conversation. To the North American this is edging toward what in his culture is an uncomfortable something—possibly sexual—which inhibits his own communication.

Yet there are cultures which restrict physical contact far more than we do. An American at a cocktail party in Java tripped over the invisible cultural ropes which mark the boundaries of acceptable behavior. He was seeking to develop a business relationship with a prominent Javanese and seemed to be doing very well. Yet, when the cocktail party ended, so apparently did a promising beginning. For the North American spent nearly six months trying to arrange a second meeting. He finally learned, through pitying intermediaries, that at the cocktail party he had momentarily placed his arm on the shoulder of the Javanese—and in the presence of other people. Humiliating! Almost unpardonable in traditional Javanese etiquette.

In this particular case, the unwitting breach was mended by a graceful apology. It is worth noting, however, that a truly cordial business relationship never did develop.

THE FIVE DIMENSIONS OF TIME

If we peel away a few layers of cultural clothing, we begin to reach almost totally unconscious reactions. Our ideas of time, for example, are deeply instilled in us when we are children. If they are contradicted by another's behavior, we react with anger, not knowing exactly why. For the businessman, five important temporal concepts are: appointment time, discussion time, acquaintance time, visiting time, and time schedules.

Anyone who has travelled abroad or dealt at all extensively with non-Americans learns that punctuality is variously interpreted. It is one thing to recognize this with the mind; to adjust to a different kind of *appointment time* is quite another.

In Latin America, you should expect to spend hours waiting in outer offices. If you bring your American interpretation of what constitutes punctuality to a Latin-American office, you will fray your temper and elevate your blood pressure. For a forty-five-minute wait is not unusual—not more unusual than a five-minute wait would be in the United States. No insult is intended, no arbitrary pecking order is being established. If, in the United States, you would not be outraged by a five-minute wait, you should not be outraged by the Latin-American's forty-five-minute delay in seeing you. The time pie is differently cut, that's all.

Further, the Latin American doesn't usually schedule individual appointments to the exclusion of other appointments. The informal clock of his upbringing ticks more slowly and he rather enjoys seeing several people on different matters at the same time. The three-ring circus atmosphere which results, if interpreted in the American's scale of time and properiety, seems to signal him to go away, to tell him that he is not being properly treated, to indicate that his dignity is under attack. Not so. The clock on the wall may look the same but it tells a different sort of time.

The cultural error may be compounded by a further miscalculation. In thc United States, a consistently tardy man is likely to be considered undependable, and by our cultural clock this is a reasonable conclusion. For you to judge a Latin American by your scale of time values is to risk a major error.

Suppose you have waited forty-five minutes and there is a man in his office, by some miracle alone in the room with you. Do you now get down to business and stop "wasting time"?

If you are not forewarned by experience or a friendly advisor, you may try to do this. And it would usually be a mistake. For , in the American culture, *discussion* is a means to an end: the deal. You try to make your point quickly, efficiently, neatly. If your purpose is to arrange some major affairs, yoru instinct is probably to settle the major issues first, leave the details for later, possibly for the technical people to work out.

For the Latin American, the discussion is a part of the spice of life. Just as he tends not to be overly concerned about reserving you your specific segment of time, he tends not as rigidly to separate business from non-business. He runs it all together and wants to make something of a social event out of what you, in your culture, regard as strictly business.

The Latin American is not alone in this. The Greek businessman, partly for the same and partly for different reasons, does not lean toward the "hit-and-run" school of business behavior, either. The Greek businessman adds to the social element, however, a feeling about what length of discussion time constitutes good faith. In America, we show good faith by ignoring the details. "Let's agree on the main points. The details will take care of themselves."

Not so the Greek. He signifies good will and good faith by what may seem to you an interminable discussion which includes every conceivable detail. Otherwise, you see, he cannot help but feel that the other man might be trying to pull the wool over his eyes. Our habit, in what we feel to be our relaxed and friendly way, of postponing details until later smacks the Greek between the eyes as a maneuver to flank him. Even if you can somehow convince him that this is not the case, the meeting must still go on a certain indefinite—but, by our standards, long—time or he will feel disquieted.

The American desire to get down to business and on with other things works to our disadvantage in other parts of the world, too; and not only in business. The head of a large, successful Japanese firm commented: "You Americans have a terrible weakness. We Japanese know about it and exploit it every chance we get. You are impatient. We have learned that if we just make you wait long enough, you'll agree to anything."

Whether this is literally true or not, the Japanese executive singled out a trait of American culture which most of us share and which, one may assume from the newspapers, the Russians have not overlooked, either.

By *acquaintance time* we mean how long you must know a man before you are willing to do business with him.

In the United States, if we know that a salesman represent a well-known, reputable company, and if we need his product, he may walk away from the first meeting with an order in his pocket. A few minutes conversation to decide matters of price, delivery, payment, model of product—nothing more is involved. In Central America, local custom does not permit a salesman to land in town, call on the customer and walk away with an order, no matter how badly your prospect wants and needs your product. It is traditional there that you must see your man at least three times before you can discuss the nature of your business.

Does this mean that the South American businessman does not recognize the merits of one product over another? Of course it doesn't. It is just that the weight of tradition presses him to do business within a circle of friends. If a product he needs is not available within his circle, he does not go outside it so much as he enlarges the circle itself to include a new friend who can supply the want. Apart from his cultural need to "feel right" about a new relationship, there is the logic of his business system. One of the realities of his life is that it is dangerous to enter into business with someone over whom you have no more than formal, legal "control." In the past decades, his legal system has not always been as firm as ours and he has learned through experience that he needs the sanctions implicit in the informal system of friendship.

Visting time involves the question of who sets the time for a visit. George Coelho, a social psychologist from India, gives an illustrative case. A U.S. businessman received this invitation from an Indian businessman: "Won't you and your family come and see us? Come anytime." Several weeks later, the Indian repeated the invitation in the same words. Each time the American replied that he would certainly like to drop in—but he never did. The reason is obvious in terms of our culture. Here "come any time" is just an expression of friendliness. You are not really expected to show up unless your host proposes a specific time. In India, on the contrary, the words are meant literally—that the host is putting himself at the disposal of his guest and really expects him to come. It is the essence of politeness to leave it to the guest to set a time at his convenience. If the guest never comes, the Indian naturally assumes that he does not want to come. Such a misunderstanding can lead to a serious rift between men who are trying to do business with each other.

Time schedules present Americans with another problem in many parts of the world. Without schedules, deadlines, priorities, and timetables, we tend to feel that our country could not run at all. Not only are they essential to getting work done, but they also play an important role in the informal communication process. Deadlines indicate priorities and priorities signal the relative importance of people and the processes they control. These are all so much a part of our lives that a day hardly passes without some reference to them. "I have to be there by 6:30." "If I don't have these plans out by 5:00 they'll be useless." "I told J. B. I'd be finished by noon tomorrow and now he tells me to drop everything and get hot on the McDermott account. What do I do now?"

In our system, there are severe penalties for not completing work on time and important rewards for holding to schedules. One's integrity and reputation are at stake.

You can imagine the fundamental conflicts that arise when we attempt to do business with people who are just as strongly oriented away from time schedules as we are toward them.

The Middle Eastern peoples are a case in point. Not only is our idea of time schedules no part of Arab life but the mere mention of a deadline to an Arab is like waving a red flag in front of a bull. In his culture, your emphasis on a deadline has the emotional effect on him that his backing you into a corner and threatening you with a club would have on you.

One effect of this conflict of unconscious habit patterns is that hundreds of American-owned radio sets are lying on the shelves of Arab radio repair shops, untouched. The Americans made the serious cross-cultural error of asking to have the repair completed by a certain time.

How do you cope with this? How does the Arab get another Arab to do anything? Every culture has its own ways of bringing pressure to get results. The usual Arab way is one which Americans avoid as "bad manners." It is needling.

An Arab businessman whose car broke down explained it this way:

> First, I go to the garage and tell the mechanic what is wrong with my car. I wouldn't want to give him the idea that I didn't know. After that, I leave the car and walk around the block. When I come back to the garage, I ask him if he has started to work yet. On my way home from lunch I stop in and ask him how things are going. When I go back to the office I stop by again. In the evening, I return and peer over his shoulder for a while. If I didn't keep this up, he'd be off working on someone else's car.

If you haven't been needled by an Arab, you just haven't been needled.

A PLACE FOR EVERYTHING

We say that there is a time and place for everything, but compared to other countries and cultures we give very little emphasis to place distinctions. Business is almost a universal value with us; it can be discussed almost anywhere, except perhaps in church. One can even talk business on the church steps going to and from the service. Politics is only slightly more restricted in the places appropriate for its discussion.

In other parts of the world, there are decided place restrictions on the discussion of business and politics. The American who is not conscious of the unwritten laws will offend if he abides by his own rather than by the local rules.

In India, you should not talk business when visiting a man's home. If you do, you prejudice your chances of ever working out a satisfactory business relationship.

In Latin America, although university students take an active interest in politics, tradition decrees that a politican should avoid political subjects when speaking on university grounds. A Latin American politician commented to anthropologist Allan Holmberg that neither he nor his fellow politicans would have dared attempt a political speech on the grounds of the University of San Marcos in Peru—as did Vice-President Nixon.

To complicate matters further, the student body of San Marcos, anticipating the visit, had voted that Mr. Nixon would not be welcome. The University Rector had issued no invitation, presumably because he expected what did, in fact, happen.

As a final touch, Mr. Nixon's interpreter was a man in full military uniform. In Latin American countries, some of which had recently overthrown military dictators, the symbolism of the military uniform could hardly contribute to a cordial atmosphere. Latin Americans need no reminder that the United States is a great military power.

Mr. Nixon's efforts were planned in the best traditions of our own culture: he hoped to improve relations through a direct, frank, and face-to-face discussion with students—the future leaders of their country. Unfortunately, this approach did not fit in at all with the culture of the host country. Of course, elements to the United States did their best to capitalize upon this cross-cultural misunderstanding. However, even Latin Americans friendly to us, while admiring the Vice President's courage, found themselves acutely embarrased by the behavior of their people and ours in the ensuing difficulties.

BEING COMFORTABLE IN SPACE

Like time and place, differing ideas of space hide traps for the uninformed. Without realizing it, almost any person raised in the United States is likely to give an unintended snub to a Latin American simply in the way we handle space relationships, particularly during conversations.

In North America, the "proper" distance to stand when talking to another adult male you do not know well is about two feet, at least in a formal business conversation. (Naturally at a cocktail party, the distance shrinks, but anything under eight to ten inches is likely to provoke an apology or an attempt to back up.)

To a Latin American, with his cultural traditions and habits, a distance of two feet seems to him approximately what five feet would to us. To him, we seem distant and cold. To us, he gives an impression of pushiness.

As soon as a Latin American moves close enough for him to feel comfortable, we feel uncomfortable and edge back. We once observed a conversation between a Latin and a North American which began at one end of a forty-foot hall. At intervals we noticed them again, finally at the other end of the hall. This rather amusing displacement had been accomplished by an almost continual series of small backward steps on the part of the American, trying unconsciously to reach a comfortable talking distance, and an equal closing of the gap by the Latin American as he attempted to reach his accustomed conversation space.

Americans in their offices in Latin America tend to keep their native acquaintances at our distance—not the Latin American's distance—by taking up a position behind a desk or typewriter. The barricade approach to communication is practiced even by old hands in Latin America who are completely unaware of its cultural significance. They know only that they are comfortable without realizing that the distance and equipment unconsciously make the Latin American uncomfortable.

HOW CLASS CHANNELS COMMUNICATION

We would be mistaken to regard the communication patterns which we observe around the world as no more than a miscellaneous collection of customs. The communication pattern of a given society is part of its total culture pattern and can only be understood in that context.

We cannot undertake here to relate many examples of communication behavior to the underlying culture of the country. For the businessman, it might be useful to mention the difficulties in the relationship between social levels and the problem of information feedback from lower to higher levels in industrial organizations abroad.

There is in Latin America a pattern of human relations and union-management relations quite different from that with which we are familiar in the United States. Everett Hagen of MIT has noted the heavier emphasis upon line authority and the lesser development of staff organizations in Latin-American plants when compared with North American counterparts. To a much greater extent than in the United States, the government becomes involved in the handling of all kinds of labor problems.

These differences seem to be clearly related to the culture and social organization of Latin America. We find there that society has been much more rigidly stratified than it has with us. As a corollary, we find a greater emphasis upon authority in family and the community.

This emphasis upon status and class distinction makes it very difficult for people of different status levels to express themselves freely and frankly in discussion and argument. In the past, the pattern has been for the man of lower status to express deference to his superior in any face-to-face contact. This is so even when everyone knows that the subordinate dislikes the superior. The culture of Latin America places a great premium upon keeping personal relations harmonious on the surface.

In the United States, we feel that it is not only desirable but natural to speak up to your superior, to tell the boss exactly what you think, even when you disagree with him. Of course, we do not always do this, but we think that we should, and we feel guilty if we fail to speak our minds frankly. When workers in our factories first get elected to local union office, they may find themselves quite self-conscious about speaking up to the boss and arguing grievances. Many of them, however, quickly learn to do it and enjoy the experience. American culture emphasizes the thrashing-out of differences in face-to-face contacts. It de-emphasizes the importance of status. As a result, we have built institutions for handling industrial disputes on the basis of the local situation, and we rely on direct discussion by the parties immediately involved.

In Latin America, where it is exceedingly difficult for people to express their differences face-to-face and where status differences and authority are much more strongly emphasized than here, the workers tend to look to a third party—the government—to take care of their problems. Though the workers have great difficulty in thrashing out their problems with management, they find no difficulty in telling government representatives their problems. And it is to their government that they look for an authority to settle their grievances with management.

Status and class also decide whether business will be done on an individual or a group basis.

In the United States, we are growing more and more accustomed to working as members of large organizations. Despite this, we still assume that there is no need to send a delegation to do a job that one capable man might well handle.

In some other parts of the world, the individual cannot expect to gain the respect necessary to accomplish this purpose, no matter how capable he is, unless he brings along an appropriate number of associates.

In the United States, we would rarely think it necessary or proper to call on a customer in a group. He might well be antagonized by the hard sell. In Japan—as an example—the importance of the occasion and of the man is measured by whom he takes along.

This practice goes far down in the business and government hierarchies. Even a university professor is likely to bring one or two retainers along on academic business. Otherwise people might think that he was a nobody and that his affairs were of little moment.

Even when a group is involved in the U.S., the head man is the spokesman and sets the tone. This is not always the case in Japan. Two young Japanese once requested an older American widely respected in Tokyo to accompany them so that they could "stand on his face." He was not expected to enter into the negotiation; his function was simply to be present as an indication that their intentions were serious.

ADJUSTMENT GOES BOTH WAYS

One need not have devoted his life to a study of various cultures to see that none of them is static. All are constantly changing and one element of change is the very fact that U.S. enterprise enters a foreign field. This is inevitable and may be constructive if we know how to utilize our knowledge. The problem is for us to be aware of our impact and to learn how to induce changes skillfully.

Rather than try to answer the general question of how two cultures interact, we will consider the key problem of personnel selection and development in two particular intercultural situations, both in Latin cultures.

One U.S. company had totally different experiences with "Smith" and "Jones" in the handling of its labor relations. The local union leaders were bitterly hostile to Smith, whereas they could not praise Jones enough. These were puzzling reactions to higher management. Smith seemed a fair-minded and understanding man; it was difficult to fathom how anyone could be bitter against him. At the same time, Jones did not appear to be currying favor by his generosity in giving away the firm's assets. To management, he seemed to be just as firm a negotiator as Smith.

The explanation was found in the two men's communication characteristics. When the union leaders came in to negotiate with Smith, he would let them state their case fully and freely—without interruption, but also without comment. When they had finished, he would say, "I'm sorry. We can't do it." He would follow this blunt statement with a brief and entirely cogent explanation of his reasons for refusal. If the union leaders persisted in their arguments, Smith would paraphrase his first statement, calmly and succinctly. In either case, the discussion was over in a few minutes. The union leaders would storm out of Smith's office complaining bitterly about the cold and heartless man with whom they had to deal.

Jones handled the situation differently. His final conclusion was the same as Smith's—but he would state it only after two or three hours of discussion. Furthermore, Jones participated actively in these discussions, questioning the union leaders for more information, relating the case in question to previous cases, philosophizing about labor relations and human rights and exchanging stories about work experience. When the discussion came to an end, the union leaders would leave the office, commenting on how warmhearted and understanding he was, and how confident they were that he would help them when it was possible for him to do so. They actually seemed more satisfied with a negative decision from Jones than they did with a hard-won concession from Smith.

This was clearly a case where the personality of Jones happened to match certain discernible requirements of the Latin American culture. It was happenstance in this case that Jones worked out and Smith did not, for by American standards both were top-flight men. Since a talent for the kind of negotiation that the Latin American considers graceful and acceptable can hardly be developed in a grown man (or perhaps even in a young one), the basic problem is one of personnel selection in terms of the culture where the candidate is to work.

The second case is more complicated because it involves much deeper intercultural adjustments. The management of the parent U.S. company concerned had learned—as have the directors of most large firms with good-sized installations overseas—that one cannot afford to have all of the top and middle-management positions manned by North Americans. It is necessary to advance nationals up the overseas-management ladder as rapidly as their abilities permit. So the nationals have to learn not only the technical aspects of their jobs but also how to function at higher levels in the organization.

Latin culture emphasizes authority in the home, church, and community. Within the organization this produces a built-in hesitancy about speaking up to one's superiors. The initiative, the acceptance of responsibility which we value in our organizations had to be stimulated. How could it be done?

We observed one management man who had done a remarkable job of building up these very qualities in his general foremen and foremen. To begin with, he stimulated informal contacts between himself and these men through social events to which the men and their wives came. He saw to it that his senior North American assistants and their wives were also present. Knowing the language, he mixed freely with all. At the plant, he circulated about, dropped in not to inspect or check up, but to joke and to break down the great barrier that existed in the local traditions between authority and the subordinates.

Next, he developed a pattern of three-level meetings. At the top, he himself, the superintendents, and the general foremen. At the middle level, the superintendents, general foremen, and foremen. Then the general foremen, foremen, and workers.

At the top level meeting, the American management chief set the pattern of encouraging his subordinates to challenge his own ideas, to come up with original thoughts. When his superintendents (also North Americans) disagreed with him, he made it clear that they were to state their objections fully. At first, the general foremen looked surprised and uneasy. They noted, however, that the senior men who argued with the boss were encouraged and praised. Timorously, with great hesitation, they began to add their own suggestions. As time went on, they more and more accepted the new convention and pitched in without inhibition.

The idea of challenging the boss with constructive new ideas gradually filtered down to the second and third level meetings. It took a lot of time and gentle handling, but out of this approach grew an extraordinary morale. The native general foremen and foremen developed new pride in themselves, accepted new responsibilities, even reached out for more. They began to work to improve their capacities and to look forward to moving up in the hierarchy.

CONFORMITY OR ADJUSTMENT?

To work with people, must we be just like them? Obviously not. If we try to conform completely, the Arab, the Latin American, the Italian, whoever he might be, finds our behavior confusing and insincere. He suspects our motive. We are expected to be different. But we are also expected to respect and accept the other people as they are. And we may, without doing violence to our own personalities, learn to communicate with them by observing the unwritten patterns they are accustomed to.

To be aware that there are pitfalls in cross-cultural dealings is the first big step forward. And to accept the fact that our convictions are in no respect more eternally "right" than someone else's is another constructive step.

Beyond these:

1. We can learn to control our so-called frankness in a culture which puts a high value on maintaining pleasant surface relations.
2. We can avoid expressing quick decisions when their utterance without a long period of polite preparation would show disrespect.
3. We can be on the lookout for the conversation patterns of nationals of whatever country we are in and accustom ourselves to closer quarters than we are used to. (This is uncomfortable at first but understanding the reason why it is important helps greatly.)
4. Where the situation demands it, we can learn to express our emotions more freely—most people find this rather exhilarating.
5. We can try to distinguish between the organizational practices which are really necessary to effectiveness and those that we employ from habit because they happen to be effective in the United States.

RESEARCH FOR ORGANIZATIONAL EFFECTIVENESS

We have outlined a point of view the individual can seek to apply in order to increase his own effectiveness. Valuable as that may be, we must recognize the limitations of an individual approach. Since each family transported overseas represents an investment of between $25,000 and $100,000 per year to the organization, the losses involved in poor selection or inadequate training can be enormous.

While no ready-made answers are now available, research can serve the organization both in *selection* and *training* of personnel.

It would be a mistake to assume that the ideal training program would fit just any administrator effectively into any given culture. We must assume that some personalities will fit more readily than others. By the time man reaches adulthood, his personality is rather solidly formed, and basic changes are difficult if not impossible to induce. It is therefore important to work to improve the selection process so that men with little chance of fitting into a foreign culture will not be sent where they are bound to fail.

Our Latin-American case of Smith and Jones is relevant here.

One who had observed Smith in his native setting should have been able to predict that he would not be effective in handling labor relations in Latin America. However, that statement is based upon the hindsight observation that there was a very obvious lack of fit between Smith's personality and the cultural requirements of his job. It remains for research men to devise schemes of observation and testing which will enable personnel men to base their selections upon criteria of personality *and* culture.

To what extent can training improve the effectiveness of individuals in intercultural communication? Training of men in overseas operations is going on all the time. So far as we know, little of it currently deals with the considerations outlined in this article. Until organizations are prepared to develop training along these lines—and support research on the effects of such training—we shall not know to what extent intercultural communications can be improved through training.

We do not mean to give the impression that behavioral scientists already have the knowledge needed regarding intercultural communication. What we have presented here is only a demonstration of the importance of the topic. We have not presented a systematic analysis of the problems of communication from culture A to culture B. We have just said in effect: "These are some of the things that are important. Watch out for them."

What more is needed? In the first place, the problem calls for a new emphasis in anthropological research. In the past, anthropologists have been primarily concerned with the *internal* pattern of a given culture. In giving attention to intercultural problems, they have examined the impact of one culture upon another. Very little attention has been given to the actual communication process between representatives of different cultures.

Much could be learned, for example, if we observed North Americans in interaction with people of another culture. We would want also to be able to interview both parties to the interaction to study how A was interpreting B and how B was interpreting A. In this way we might discover points of friction and miscommunication whose existence we now do not even suspect. Such studies, furthermore, would provide systematic knowledge much more useful than the fragments provided in this article.

Dominant and Variant Value Orientations

FLORENCE ROCKWOOD KLUCKHOHN

No nursing assessment is complete without an analysis of the patient's value system. What does the patient believe about health and illness, what does he understand about disease causation and treatment? Does the patient believe that his disease was caused by an act of God? Does he believe that disease is an accident of nature or that it is something over which he has some control? Does the patient believe that cure is possible through an act of will; through the application of scientific principles; or through dependence upon God's will?

These questions relate to what Florence Kluckhohn terms dominant and variant value orientations. What a person believes and values affects his behavior. The following article may be difficult reading—but the gains are worth the effort. When the patient and the nurse do not hold the same value systems, conflicting communication and goals will occur. The American nurse, educated in the United States, falls within the "Old Yankee" classification of value systems. Amer-

From *Personality in Nature, Society, and Culture* (2nd ed.), Clyde Kluckhohn and Henry A. Murray, Editors (New York: Alfred A. Knopf, Inc., 1953) pp. 342-57. Reprinted by permission of the author.

Note: A more complete version of the theory and method of testing can be found in *Variations in Value Orientations* by Florence R. Kluckhohn, Fred L. Strodbeck, et al., published in 1961 by Row Peterson and Company, and now being republished by the Greenwood Press. Elmsford, New York.

ican nurses are future-oriented, belong to a doing-oriented profession, are individualistic in decision-making but lineally oriented in the health institution, believe that disease is controllable, and view the human being as neither good nor evil, but ill. When the patient holds the same values, nurse-patient interactions will proceed positively. The problem lies with nurse-patient interaction across value systems.

When the nurse adds value orientations to her nursing assessment, her knowledge and understanding of the patient increases.

For all those concerned with the lives of individuals and the problems which arise in those lives there has long been a question—even an argument—as to how much the individual is a product of his biological heritage and how much the result of environmental forces. That either a strictly biological or an over-simply formulated environmental theory of human behavior is absurdly one-sided most of us have long ago accepted. Yet most of us also know that we are really only at the beginning of the time-consuming and arduous process from which we hope to derive an understanding of that infinitely complicated interplay of biological, psychological, social, and other factors which create the personality and character structure of individuals. We still display a tendency to concentrate on certain factors and exclude others. Some are too much given to interpretations in strictly psychological terms, some too eager to use only the conceptual lenses provided by the sociologist, the anthropologist, or the economist, and others equally zealous with still other approaches.

Today the awareness is growing—rapidly growing—that anything like a full understanding of the concrete situations in which we see individuals requires a use of the explanatory concepts of more than one discipline and requires their use in other ways than an occasional "borrowing" to account for the extraneous. The goal of an integration of our several approaches to a study of human behavior and social stituations is clearly before us and recognized as a goal, yet no one can rightly claim that we are close to achieving it.

One specific example of this growing interest in the multiple rather than the unitary approach to individual and social problems is found in the current and frequent linkage of the terms "culture" and "personality." The practical reflection of this we find in the frequent queries of many in the fields of education, social work, colonial administration, and industry as to what a knowledge of cultural factors offers them for a better understanding of the situations and the individuals with which they must deal. Even clinical psychologists and psychiatrists, whose theories have necessarily centered upon the psychological processes of the individual, are asking what the effect of varying cultural patterns upon the actions and motives of individuals may be.

Some real progress has been made, especially in the last decade or so, in bringing together psychological and socio-cultural theories. For those interested in a very brief sketch of the history of this development we would recommend Dr. Ralph Linton's introduction to Dr. Abram Kardiner's *The Psychological Frontiers of Society* [I].

Illustrative of the kind of conceptual integration which has to date been achieved, Linton points to the concept of "basic personality" which he himself and Dr. Kardiner developed in their collaborative work. Basic personality, he states, is a configuration involving several different elements. It rests upon the following postulates:

> 1. That the individual's early experiences exert a lasting effect upon his personality, especially upon the development of his projective system.
> 2. That similar experiences will tend to produce similar personality configurations in the individuals who are subjected to them.
> 3. That the techniques which the members of any society employ in the care and rearing of children are culturally patterned and will tend to be similar, although never identical, for various families within the society.
> 4. That the culturally patterned techniques for the care and rearing of children differ from one society to another.
>
> If these postulates are correct, and they seem to be supported by a wealth of evidence, it follows:
> 1. That the members of any given society will have many elements of early experience in common.
> 2. That as a result of this they will have many elements of personality in common.
> 3. That since the early experience of individuals differs from one society to another, the personality norms for various societies will also differ.
>
> The *basic personality type* for any society is that personality configuration which is shared by the bulk of the society's members as a result of the early experiences which they have in common. It does not correspond to the total personality of the individual but rather to the projective systems or, in different phraseology, the value-attitude systems which are basic to the individual's personality configuration. Thus the same basic

personality type may be reflected in many different forms of behavior and may enter into many different total personality configurations. [I, pp. vi–viii]

The studies of various other anthropologists and the collaborative work many of them have done with psychologists, psychiatrists, and sociologists have gone far in demonstrating many of the relationships between individual desires and group experiences—between culture and personality. Yet, for all of the valuable insights produced and the considerable progress thus far achieved, there have been some severe and—in the opinion of the writer—justified criticisms of many of the facile conclusions drawn by some anthropologists. Especially in some of the recent interpretations of so-called national character structure, one notes a repeated tendency to derive highly generalized and far sweeping conclusions from a few specific items of culture content. Sociologists and psychologists alike have cavilled at the apparent ignoring of interaction processes by some anthropologists and at the too deterministic effects often claimed for cultural factors.

Much of the difficulty in all attempts to use the cultural anthropologists' concepts and data arise from an absence of a systematic theory of cultural variation and from the tendency of most anthropologists to rely too much upon mere empirical generalizations. The most casual observer is aware that the customs of different societies vary. He knows, too, that the behavior patterns of individuals within a given society are often markedly different. Indeed, when dealing with variation at this level one cannot but be acutely conscious of the wide range of "individual differences." But it is not this plethora of specific content which is of the most critical importance if the aim is to understand better the relationship of cultural factors to either the structuring of social groups or the personalities of the individuals who comprise the social groups. It is rather the generalized meanings or values which should be the major, or at least the first, concern. *Specific patterns of behavior insofar as they are influenced by cultural factors (and few are not so influenced) are the concrete expressions reflecting generalized meanings or values. And to the extent that the individual personality is a product of training in a particular cultural tradition it is also at the generalized value level that one finds the most significant differences.*

As Gregory Bateson has remarked: "The human individual is endlessly simplifying, organizing, and generalizing his own view of his own environment; he constantly imposes his own constructions and meanings; these constructions and meanings (are) characteristic of one culture as over against another [2]." Or, as Clyde Kluckhohn stated: "There is a 'philosophy' behind the way of life of every individual and of every relatively homogeneous group at any given point in their histories [3]."

The writer agrees with these and many similar statements made by other anthropologists which emphasize the importance of "value orientations" in the lives of individuals and groups of individuals [4]. There is in many of them, however, too much stress—implied when not actually stated—upon the unitary character of value orientations. Variation for the same individual when he is playing different roles and variation between whole groups of persons within a single society are not adequately accounted for. More important still, the emphasis upon the uniqueness of the variable value systems or different societies ignores the fact of the universality of human problems and the correlate fact that human societies have found for some problems approximately the same answers. Yet certainly it is only within a frame of reference which deals with universals that variation can be understood. Without it, it is not possible to deal systematically with either the problem of similarity and difference as between the value systems of different societies or the question of variant values within societies.

Human behavior mirrors at all times an intricate blend of the universal and the variable. The universals and variations are of many kinds. All human beings have many and significant biological similarities as members of a particular species—*homo sapiens*—yet variability within the species is great. We frequently note both the similarities and differences which are psychological.

The problem of the dominant and variant in cultural patterning can, of course, be approached in different ways. Precisely which way will depend upon the specific type of investigation being made. The aim of the approach of this paper is a conceptual scheme which will permit a systematic ordering of cultural value orientations within the framework of common human—universal—problems. It is only when we have delineated the central types of value orientations and the ranges of possible variability in them that we can make systematic comparisons of either single orientations or the total *value orientation profiles* of whole societies or parts of societies.

The first fundamental assumption upon which the conceptual scheme is based is: *There is a limited number of basic human problems for which all peoples at all times and in all places must find some solution.* The five common human problems tentatively singled out as those of key importance can be stated in the form of questions:

1. What are the *innate predispositions* of man? (Basic human nature)
2. What is the relation of *man to nature?*

3. What is the significant *time* dimension?
4. What is the valued *personality type?*
5. What is the dominant modality of the *relationship of man to other men?*

The problems as stated in these questions are regarded as constant; they arise inevitably out of the human situation. The solutions found for them are variable but not limitlessly so. It is the second major assumption of the conceptual scheme that *the variability in solutions is variability within a range of possible solutions.* The limits of variability suggested as a testable conceptualization are the three point ranges for each of the main orientations given in TABLE XXXIX. Nothing mystical is claimed for the number *three*, but as will be seen in the following explanations, such a breakdown seems, in almost all cases, to be both logically adequate and empirically sound.

TABLE XXXIX HUMAN PROBLEMS AND TYPE SOLUTIONS

Innate Predispositions:	Evil (mutable or immutable)	Neither good nor bad mutable or immutable)	Good (mutable or immutable)
Man's Relation to Nature:	Man subjugated to nature	Man in nature	Man over nature
Time Dimension:	Past	Present	Future
Valued Personality Type:	Being	Being-in-Becoming	Doing
Modality of Relationship:	Lineal	Collateral	Individualistic

To the question of what innate human nature is, there are the three logical divisions of evil, neither good nor evil (or mixed), and good. And such, in fact, seem to be the distinctions which have been made by societies. Variation within this range is, of course, possible. Human nature can be regarded as evil and unalterable or evil and perfectible. It can be good and unalterable or good and corruptible. It can be viewed as neither good nor evil and treated as invariant or as subject to influence. This kind of variability, however, falls within the basic threefold classification and is probably a result of the relationship of the human-nature orientation to other orientations.

Illustrations of these differences in the definition of innate predispositions are easily found. We have only to look about us to recognize that there is considerable variability in our present day American conception of human nature. The orientation we inherited from Puritan ancestors, and still strong in many of us, is that human nature is basically evil but perfectible. Constant control and discipline of the self are essential if any real goodness is to be achieved and maintained, and the danger of regression is always present. But some in our society today—perhaps a growing number—are inclined to the more tolerant view that human nature is a mixture of the good and the bad. These would say that control and effort are certainly needed, but lapses can be understood and need not always be severely condemned. Such a definition of basic human nature would appear to be a somewhat more common one among the peoples of the world—both literate and nonliterate—than the view we have held in our own historical past. Whether there are any total societies given to the definition of human nature as *immutably good* is to be doubted. The position is, however, a possible one and should be found ever present as an alternative definition within societies.

The three-point range of variation in the *man-nature* relationship—that of Man Subjugated to Nature, Man In Nature, and Man Over Nature—is too well known from the work of philosophers and culture historians to need a detailed explanation. Mere illustration will demonstrate the differences.

Spanish-American culture as I have known it in the American Southwest illustrates well the Man Subjugated to Nature position. To the typical Spanish-American sheep-raiser in that region there is little or nothing which can be done if a storm comes to damage his range lands or destroy his flocks. He simply accepts the inevitable as the inevitable. His attitude toward illness and death is the same fatalistic attitude. "If it is the Lord's will that I die I shall die" is the way he expresses it. Many a Spanish-American has been known to refuse the help of any doctor because of this attitude.

Another way of phrasing the *man-nature* relationship is to regard all natural forces and man himself as one harmonious whole. One is but an extension of the other, and both are needed to make the whole. Such was the attitude frequently found as the dominant one in China in the past centuries.

A third way of viewing this relationship is that of Man Against—or Over—Nature. According to this view, which is clearly the one characteristic of Americans, natural forces are something to be overcome and put to the use of human beings. We span our rivers with bridges, blast through our mountains to make tunnels, make lakes where none existed, and do a thousand and one other things to exploit nature and make it serve our human needs. In general this means that we have an orientation to life which is that of overcoming obstacles. And it is difficult for us to understand the kind of people who accept the obstacle and give in to it or even the people who stress the harmonious oneness of man and nature.

The possible cultural phrasings of the *man in time* problem breaks easily into the three point range of Past, Present and Future. Far too little attention has been given to this problem and its phrasings. Meaningful cultural differences have been lost sight of in the too sweeping and too generalized view that folk peoples have no time sense, and no need of one, whereas urbanized and industrial peoples must have one. Whether days are regarded as sunrise to sundown wholes or as split into hours and minutes, and whether or not a clock is deemed a useful culture object are not the critically important criteria for a consideration of the orientation to time.

Spengler had quite another order of fact in mind than this when he made, in his quite profound discussion of "time" in the *Decline of the West*, this emphatic and categorical statement: "It is by the meaning that it intuitively attaches to time that one culture is differentiated from another [5]." Time and Destiny were what were being related in Spengler's conception. For the most part his concern was with the twofold division of orientations into those which were the timeless a-historic present and the ultra-historical projection into the future. Always on the plane of the macroscopic and concerned with directionality as a cyclical unfolding, he apparently did not feel a need to deal with the problem of the traditionalistic or past orientation which was so important a part of Max Weber's treatment of moral authority. The threefold division proposed for the cultural orientation schema has, therefore, its similarity to Spengler's conception in the distinction between a timeless, traditionless, future-ignoring present and a realizable future. It differs in that it also differentiates from these an orientation which looks to the traditions of the past either as something to be maintained or as something to be recaptured. There is in the conception as here phrased an aspect of the orientation which is relative to the standards and norms of authority which is not explicitly included in Spengler's conception.

Obviously all societies at all times must deal with all the three time-problems. All have some conception of the past, all have a present, and all give some kind of attention to the future time-dimension. They differ, however, in their emphasis on past, present, or future at a given period, and a very great deal can be told about the particular society or part of a society being studied, much about the direction of change within it can be predicted, with a knowledge of where that emphasis is.

Illustrations of these different emphases are also easily found. Spanish-Americans, whom we have described as having the attitude that man is a victim of natural forces, are also a people who emphasize present time. They pay little attention to what has happened in the past, and regard the future as a vague and most unpredictable period. Planning for the future or hoping that the future will be better than either present or past simply is not their way of life. In dealing with Spanish-Americans one must always take into account the fact that they have quite a different time sense from our own. Too often, we, who are in the habit of making definite appointments for two or five o'clock and expect to keep and have them kept, are baffled by the Spanish-Americans to whom two or five o'clock means little or nothing. For an appointment made for two o'clock he may arrive at any time between one and five o'clock, or, most likely, he will not arrive at all. Something else which interests him more may well have turned up to absorb his attention.

China of past generations, and to some extent still, was a society which put its main emphasis upon past time. Ancestor worship and a strong family tradition were both expressions of this Past Time orientation. So also was the Chinese attitude that nothing new ever happened in the present or would happen in the future. It had all happened before in the far distant past. Thus it was that the proud American who thought he was showing some Chinese a steamboat for the first time was quickly put in his place by the remark: "Our ancestors had such a boat two thousand years ago." Many modern European countries also tended to stress the past. Even England—insofar as it has been dominated by an aristocracy and traditionalism—has voiced this emphasis. Indeed, one of the chief differences between ourselves and the English is to be found in our somewhat varying attitudes toward time. We have difficulty in understanding the respect the English have for tradition, and they do not appreciate our disregard for it.

Americans, more than most people of the world, place emphasis upon the future—a future which we anticipate to be "bigger and better." This does not mean we have no regard for the past or fail to give thought to the present. But it certainly is true that no current generation of Americans ever wants to be called "old-fashioned." We do not consider the ways of the past to be good just because they are past, and we are seldom content with the present. This makes of us a people who place a high value on change.

The fourth of the common human problems is called the *Valued Personality Type.* The range of variation in this case yields the Being, the Being-in-Becoming, and the Doing orientations. Since it is assumed that all the orientations are an aspect of the action and motivational systems of the individual personalities, *Valued Personality Type* is not the happiest of terms for designating this particular range of them. For the time being, however, we shall retain the term.

These orientations have been derived for the most part from the distinction long made by philosophers between Being and Becoming. Indeed, to a marked degree, the three-way distinction is in accord with the classification of personality components made by the philosopher Charles Morris—the Dionysian, the Apollonian, and the Promethean. The abstractly conceived component which he labels the *Dionysian*—the personality component type which releases and indulges existing desires—is somewhat what is meant by the Being orientation. His *Apollonian* component—the component type that is self-contained and controls itself through a meditation and detachment that bring understanding—is to some extent the Being-in-Becoming. His active, striving *Promethean* component is similar to the Doing orientation [6].

The accordance is, however, far from complete. As used in this schema the terms Being and Becoming, now made into the three-point range of Being, Being-in-Becoming, and Doing, are much more narrowly defined than has been the custom of philosophers. Furthermore, the view here is that these orientations vary independently relative to those which deal with the relation of man to nature, to time and innate predispositions. The tendency of the philosophers, writing with different aims, has been to treat these several types of orientations as relatively undifferentiated clusters.

The essence of the Being orientation is that it stresses the spontaneous expression of what is conceived to be "given" in the personality. The orientation is, as compared with the Being-in-Becoming or Doing, essentially *non*developmental. It might even be phrased as a spontaneous expression of impulses and desires; yet care must be taken not to make this interpretation a too literal one. In no society, as Clyde Kluckhohn has commented, does one ever find a one-to-one relationship between the desired and the desirable. The concrete behavior of individuals in complex situations and the moral codes governing that behavior usually reflect all the orientations simultaneously. A stress upon the "isness" of the personality and a spontaneous expression of that "isness" is not pure license as we can easily see if we turn our attention to a society or segments of a society in which the Being orientation is dominant. Mexican society, for example, is clearly one in which the Being orientation is dominant. Their wide-range patterning of *Fiesta* activities alone shows this. Yet never in the *Fiesta* or other patterns of spontaneity is there pure impulse gratification. The value demands of other of the orientations—the relational orientation, the conception of human nature as being good and evil and in need of control and others—all make for codes which restrain individuals in very definite ways.

The Being-in-Becoming orientation shares with the Being a great concern with what the human being is rather than what he can accomplish, but here the similarity ends. In the Being-in-Becoming orientation the idea of development so little stressed in the Being orientation is paramount.

Erich Fromm's conception of "the spontaneous activity of the total integrated personality" is close to the Being-in-Becoming type. "By activity," he states, "we do not mean 'doing something' but rather the quality of the creative activity which can operate in one's emotional, intellectual, and sensuous experiences and in one's will as well. One premise of this spontaneity is the acceptance of the total personality and the elimination of the split between reason and nature [7]." A less favorably prejudiced and, for our purposes, a more accurately limited statement would be: the Being-in-Becoming orientation emphasizes self-realization—self-development—of all aspects of the self as an integrated whole.

The Doing orientation is so characteristically the one dominantly stressed in American society that there is little need for an extensive definition. Its most distinguishing feature is its demand for action in the sense of accomplishment and in accord with standards which are conceived as being external to the acting individual. Self-judgment as well as the judgment of others is largely by means of measurable accomplishment through action. What does the individual do, what can he, or will he, accomplish are almost always primary questions in our scale of appraisal of persons. "Getting things done" and finding ways "to do something" about any and all situations are stock American phrases. Erich Fromm also recognizes this orientation as separable from that which he defines in his concept of spontaneity and which we have called the Being-in-Becoming, but he seems to view it as mainly compulsive. With this I cannot agree. Many persons in our society who follow patterns in accord with the Doing orientation are compulsive; many are not. Conformity, which is essential in all societies, whatever the arrangement of their orientations, should not be so much and so often confounded with compulsiveness.

The fifth and last of the common human problems treated in this conceptual scheme is the definition of man's relation to other men. This orientation, the *relational*, has three sub-divisions: the Lineal, the Collateral, and the Individualistic.

Sociologists have long used various types of dichotomies to differentiate homogeneous folk societies from the more complex urban societies. *Gemeinschaft-gesellschaft*, traditionalistic—rational-legal, mechanical-organic solidarity, or simply rural-urban—are the most familiar of the several paired terms. Anthropologists, who have for the most part studied *gemeinschaft* or folk peoples, have frequently in their analyses of kinship structure or social organization made much of the difference between lineage and a lateral extension of relationships.

The distinctions being made here obviously owe much to the concepts used in both these fields, but they are not identical with those of either field. The Lineal, Collateral, and Individualistic relational principles are analytical elements in total relational systems and are not to be confused with categories descriptive of concrete systems.

It is in the nature of the case that all societies—all groups—must give some attention to all three principles. Individual autonomy cannot be and is not ignored by the most extreme type of *gemeinschaft* society. Collaterality is found in all societies. The individual is not a human being outside a group and one kind of group emphasis is that put upon laterally extended relationships. These are the immediate relationships in time and place. All societies must also pay some attention to the fact that individuals are biologically and culturally related to each other through time. This is to say that there is always a Lineal principle in relationships which is derived from age and generational differences and cultural tradition. The fundamental question is always that of emphasis.

There will always be variability in the primacy and nature of goals according to which of the three principles is stressed. If the individualistic principle is dominant and the other two interpreted in terms of it—as is the case in the United States—individual goals will have primacy over the goals of either the Collateral or Lineal group. When the Collateral principle is dominant, the goals—or welfare—of the laterally extended group have primacy for all individuals. The group in this case is viewed as being moderately independent of other similar groups and the question of continuity through time is not critical. Where the Lineal principle is most heavily stressed it is again group goals which are of primary concern to individuals, but there is the additional factor that an important one of those goals is continuity through time. Both continuity and ordered positional succession are of great importance when Lineality dominates the *relational* system. Spanish-American society has been, until recently, one with a relatively strong Lineal stress, combined with a strong second order Collaterality.

How continuity and ordered positional succession are achieved in a Lineal *relational* system is separate from the principle as such. It does in fact seem to be the case that the most successful way of maintaining a stress on Lineality is through mechanisms which are either actual hereditary ones based upon biological relatedness or ones which are assimilated to a kinship system. The English, for example, maintained such an emphasis into the present time by consistently moving successful members of its more individualistic middle class into the established peerage system. Other societies have found other but similar mechanisms.

Thus far in the discussion of the major orientations the aim has been to show that different societies make different selections among possible solutions of common human problems. They raise to dominant position some one of the alternative principles. However, at no time has it been stated or implied that any society will or can ignore any of the dimensions. On the contrary, it is a fundamental proposition of this conceptual approach that all dimensions of all orientations *not only are but must be* present at all times in the pattern structure of every society.

However important it is to know what is dominant in a society at a given time, we shall not go far toward the understanding of the dynamics of that society without paying careful heed to the variant orientations. That there be individuals and whole groups of individuals who live in accordance with patterns which express variant rather than the dominantly stressed orientations is, it is maintained, essential to the maintenance of the society. *Variant values, are, therefore, not only permitted but actually required.* It has been the mistake of many in the social sciences, and of many in the field of practical affairs as well, to treat all behavior and certain aspects of motivation which do not accord with the dominant values as some kind of deviance. It is urged that we cease to confuse the deviant who by his behavior calls down the sanctions of his group with the variant who is accepted and frequently required as far as the total social system is concerned. This is especially true in a society such as ours, where beneath the surface of what has so often been called our compulsive conformity, there lies a wide range of variation. The dynamic interplay of the dominant and the variant is one of the outstanding features of American society, but as yet it has been little analyzed or understood.

Illustrations of variant value orientations, whether of individuals or whole groups, are numerous. Let us look at these three kinds: *ethnic difference* of which the United States has had, and still has, so much; *class difference; role difference* as it is seen in the role of the American woman.

The usual tendency of most observers has been either to view all ethnic groups as one undifferentiated whole or, with a concern for understanding better the problems of particular groups, to seek out the quite specific ways in which they differ. Attention is given to the kind of parental authority and to the attitude they have toward women, or perhaps we delve into the type of child-training patterns they follow. These specific patterns are of course, important; but it is obvious that knowing them all is in most cases impossible. Furthermore, when there is no general framework within which to consider the specific differences noted, there develops so frequently a tendency to attribute too much to single items of cultural content.

We could know many such concrete patterns followed by the Spanish-Americans in the Southwest and still not know why after one hundred years within the borders of the United States their way of life has changed so little until very recently. We can know and have known many such patterns and yet are forced to admit that understanding between Anglo-Americans and Spanish-Americans is not, even now, very great.

When, however, we look to fundamental differences in value orientations we are led quickly to this proposition: The slow rate of assimilation of Spanish-Americans (and more recent Mexican immigrants), and the low level of understanding as well, are in large part attributable to a wide disparity in *all* the major orientations of Anglo-Americans and Spanish-Americans.

Illustrations of most of the Spanish-American orientations have already been given singly. Let us now take them as a whole system and again quickly compare them to the system of orientations dominantly stressed in American society. Where the Anglo-American stresses Individualism, the Spanish-American puts his primary emphasis upon a combination of the Lineal and the Collateral. The semi-feudal *patron-peon* system of Mexicans, both in the United States and in Mexico, has neither permitted nor required very much independent behavior of most people. Or, to phrase this another way, whereas the Anglo-American is quite systematically trained for independent behavior, the Spanish-American or Mexican is trained for dependence.

The American dominant *time* orientation has been noted to be Future, that of the Spanish-Americans, Present. We show a vague awareness of this difference when we so often refer to Mexicans in general as being a *mañana* people. Yet how very much bound by our own cultural values we are when we interpret *manana* to mean that a Mexican will always put off until tomorrow what should be done today. Tomorrow in a highly specific sense is meaningless to the Spanish-American or Mexican. He lives in a timeless present, and as one Mexican scholar phrased it: "The Mexican never puts off until tomorrow what can be done *only* today."

Consider, too, the vast difference between the Spanish-American Being orientation and the American emphasis upon Doing or accomplishing. Doing things in the name of accomplishment is not usual Spanish-American behavior. That which "is" is in large part taken for granted and considered as something to be enjoyed rather than altered.

Our own and the Spanish-Americans' definition of the *man-nature* relationship are likewise poles apart. We set out to conquer, overcome, and exploit nature; they accept the environment with a philosophical calm bordering on the fatalistic. And seldom in Spanish-American culture does one find evidence of our own historical view of human nature as Evil but Perfectible. Their view would appear to be much more that of human nature as a Mixture of the Good and Bad.

With such differences as these it is not a cause for wonder that Anglo-American educators, social workers, politicians, and a host of others have been both deeply frustrated and quite unsuccessful in their many attempts either to alter rapidly the Spanish-American way of life or adjust Anglo-American values to it. Nor is it strange that the understanding between Anglo- and Spanish-Americans in an area (New Mexico and Arizona) where each group constitutes approximately a half of the total population has been inadequate throughout a whole century.

This highly dramatic and most extreme illustration of cultural variation within our own borders tells us a great deal if only we look at it in terms of major value orientations instead of always considering particular and specific bits of behavior. The specific to be very meaningful, we repeat, must be viewed as an item in the wider context of value orientations.

Generalizing this conception to all such groups as the Spanish-American we would first hypothesize that *the rate and degree of assimilation of any ethnic group into general dominant American culture will in large part depend upon the degree of goodness of fit of the group's own basic value orientations with those of dominant American culture.*

Class differences have greatly concerned American social scientists in the last two decades. The best known studies of the class structure of the United States are those of W. Lloyd Warner and his associates, but there are also many others with different points of view and in which conclusions very different from those of the Warner group are reached. From all the studies we have learned much that Americans have been unwilling to admit or discuss in past years. We know that there are great differences between the classes in attitudes toward education and politics, in association memberships, in family life, in occupational interests and opportunities, in reading habits, in recreational interests; and a host of other things.

Yet in spite of all the differences observed and recorded, there is a tendency in all the studies to assume that all the variation is variation on the same value theme—the so-called American Creed. What is remarked is that the behavior and attitudes of some classes are harmoniously in tune with the generalized creed, whereas those of other classes are off in pitch and limited in range. That the value themes themselves might be different is seldom suggested.

But according to the conceptual scheme of the dominant and variant in cultural orientations, it is assumed at the start that there is a dominant class—in the case of the United States, the middle class—in which adherence to dominant values is marked, but also that there are other classes which hold to variant values in much of what they do and believe. As I have suggested elsewhere, the observed behavior of an upper class in an old and declining community shows an adherence to lineality rather than individualism, to past time more than future, and to Being or Being-in-Becoming rather than to Doing personalities. Also in some parts of the lower class—a class so heterogeneous and diffuse that it should be "classes" and not just "class"—Present Time and Being orientations are often combined with either Individualism or Collaterality.

There has not been sufficient work done to date to state with certainty that this different approach will provide a more accurate knowledge and appraisal of class differences. One study now in progress—a study of the occupational aspirations of a large group of high school boys in a metropolitan community—shows some promise of demonstrating the existence of value orientation differences between classes and segments of classes [8]. In another study just completed by Dr. Charles McArthur it has been shown that, on the average, public and private school boys give predictably different responses to the pictures in the Murray and Morgan Thematic Apperception Test [9]. For example, on the assumption that in a public school boys are predominantly middle class and hence Future Time and Doing oriented, while private school boys—especially those of certain selected schools—are predominantly upper class with Past Time and either a Being or Being-in-Becoming orientation, these two predictions were made as to the variability of responses to the first picture of the test (a small boy is seated before a table on which there lies a violin; the subject is asked to invent a story about him):

1. That more public school boys (now students in a large university) will tell stories to the violin picture in which the parent demands work from the child.
2. That more private school boys will tell violin stories in which the music lesson is seen by the child as a way to create beauty and/or express or develop himself.

These predictions, and twelve others similar in type but different in content, were borne out by McArthur's data. And, as he himself said: "They constituted a neat demonstration that the attitudes of individuals, as measured by one of the psychologist's best projective tests of personality, can be predicted from a knowledge of the person's sub-cultural orientations profile."

The role of the woman in the United States is as little understood for its variant character as are some of the differences in social classes. Although it is frequently stated that the feminine role is poorly defined and full of contradictions, it has not been noted that the behavior expected of women in the wife-mother role is relative to value orientations which are markedly different from the dominant American values that are so well expressed in the man's occupational role.

In his occupational role the Man—ideally at least—is expected to be autonomous and independent, whereas from the woman as a wife and mother we all expect a subordination of individualistic goals to those of the family as a group. Man's occupational role is also an action-oriented one which expresses well the Doing orientation, while in woman's role it is expected that much more attention will be given to all those things intellectual, aesthetic, and moral which busy men so often define as the nice but non-essential embroidery of American life. It is, in other words, more of the Being-in-Becoming orientation that women are supposed to adhere to. As for the *Time* orientation it is again man's role which most fully expresses Americans' dominant *future* emphasis. For the most part, daughters and wives are limited to a vicarious participation in the goals of future promise. The glory which comes from mounting success is largely a man's glory, the light from which is, for women, merely reflective.

Differences such as these are both considerable and troublesome in a society which theoretically stands for an equality of the sexes. When one studies carefully the history of the feminine role it becomes very clear that a central issue for many years has been woman's demand for the right to participate more fully in all those activities in which *dominant* American values are expressed.

In recent years the issue has become the more acute because of the kind of education the women of today receive. Girls are no longer trained in markedly different ways or for different things than boys are. Throughout childhood and youth the girl child goes to school with boys and is taught very much as they are taught. From babyhood on, she learns the ways of being independent and autonomous, and she is expected to know how to look after herself all through adolescence and beyond—forever if need be. The hope is expressed, of course, that she will not have to remain independent and will not, therefore, need to use much of what she has learned. Instead, and this is the truly great problem, she is expected, upon her marriage, or certainly after children are born, to give her attention to all those things which are defined as feminine and for which she has not been well trained at all. It is not to be wondered that the strains in the feminine role are numerous and make for serious personality difficulties in many women.

In other instances of variant roles the strains are fewer. The man who chooses to be a withdrawn scholar or an artist may often be made to feel that he is outside the main stream of life, but it is doubtful that he is subject to as many doubts about the value of what he does as are many women. In the main this is because he is creative, whereas the intellectual and aesthetic interests of women have been, to date, chiefly appreciative.

There is, of course, much more value variation within our own or any other social system than these few illustrations indicate. The varying roles any individual plays at different times and places may be, and often are, different in the value orientations they express. No individual any more than any whole society can live always in all situations in accord with patterns which allow for expression of only a single dimension of the orientations. One can also note many shifts of emphasis in the range of one orientation or another as between the different historical time periods of a social system. Indeed, whatever the type of problem or the situation one may choose for study, variations in value orientations are certain to be found. Thus we repeat: If a knowledge of major cultural value orientations is essential to the understanding of social situations and individual personalities (and I would say it certainly is), it is also necessary to know the variant value orientations and their relation to the dominant ones.

REFERENCES

1. Kardiner, Abram: *The Psychological Frontiers of Society* (New York, Columbia University Press, 1945).
2. Bateson, Gregory: "Cultural Determinants of Personality," in J. McV. Hunt (ed.): *Personality and the Behavior Disorders* (New York, Ronald Press, 1944), Vol. 2, p. 273.
3. Kluckhohn, Clyde: "Values and Value Orientations in the Theory of Action," in Talcott Parsons and Edward A. Shils (eds.): *Toward a General Theory of Action* (Cambridge, Harvard University Press, 1951), p. 409.
4. Kluckhohn, Ibid., p. 411, defines value orientation as follows: "a generalized and organized conception, influencing behavior, of nature, of man's place in it, of man's relation to man, and of the desirable and non-desirable as they may relate to man-environment and interhuman relations."

5. Spengler, Oswald: *The Decline of the West*, tr. Charles F. Atkinson (New York, Knopf, 1926-8).
6. Morris, Charles: *Paths of Life* (New York, Harpers, 1942), esp. chap. II.
7. Fromm, Erich: *Escape from Freedom* (New York, Farrar and Rhinehart, 1941).
8. This project is sponsored by the Harvard University Laboratory of Social Relations and is under the direction of Professors Samuel A. Stouffer and Talcott Parsons and the writer.
9. McArthur, Charles: Cultural Values as Determinants of Imaginal Productions, unpublished Ph.D. thesis, Harvard University, 1952.

Continuities and Discontinuities in Cultural Conditioning

RUTH BENEDICT

A standard part of any nursing assessment includes information on the patient's past medical and hospitalization history. This information can direct the nurse to further assessment of the patient's socialization into the patient role. Patients do not go to school to learn to be patients.. They are socialized, rather than educated, to their role. The patient learns how to be a patient through interaction with every member of the health team. The patient learns, directly or indirectly, what is expected of him as a patient. Patients learn where they are to go, what they are to do, what decisions they can make, and what questions they are allowed to ask from nurses, physicians, other patients, and other members of the health team.

Patients are culturally conditioned into the patient role. But is that conditioning always continuous? Do all nurses or all health professionals agree on what is expected behavior on the part of the patient? Are all patients socialized to becoming a patient, being a patient, or becoming a discharged patient on a continuous scale? The discontinuity of cultural conditioning of patients within and across cultures has many of the same features as those discussed by Benedict for other ascribed social roles.

Reprinted by special permission of the William Alanson Whyte Psychiatric Foundation, Inc. From *Psychiatry* 1 (1938):161-67.

All cultures must deal in one way or another with the cycle of growth from infancy to adulthood. Nature has posed the situation dramatically: on the one hand, the new born baby, physiologically vulnerable, unable to fend for itself, or to participate of its own initiative in the life of the group, and, on the other, the adult man or woman. Every man who rounds out his human potentialities must have been a son first and a father later and the two roles are physiologically in great contrast; he must first have been dependent upon others for his very existence and later he must provide such security for others. This discontinuity in the life cycle is a fact of nature and is inescapable. Facts of nature, however, in any discussion of human problems, are ordinarily read off not at their bare minimal but surrounded by all the local accretions of behavior to which the student of human affairs has become accustomed in his own culture. For that reason it is illuminating to examine comparative material from other societies in order to get a wider perspective on our own special accretions. The anthropologist's role is not to question the facts of nature, but to insist upon the interposition of a middle term between "nature" and "human behavior"; his role is to analyse that term, to document local man-made doctorings of nature and to insist that these doctorings should not be read off in any one culture as nature itself. Although it is a fact of nature that the child becomes a man, the way in which this transition is effected varies from one society to another, and no one of these particular cultural bridges should be regarded as the "natural path to maturity.

From a comparative point of view our culture goes to great extremes in emphasizing contrasts between the child and the adult. The child is sexless, the adult estimates his virility by his sexual activities; the child must be protected from the ugly facts of life, the adult must meet them without psychic catastrophe; the child must obey, the adult must command this obedience. These are all dogmas of our culture, dogmas which in spite of the facts of nature, other cultures commonly do not share. In spite of the physiological contrasts between child and adult these are cultural accretions.

It will make the point clearer if we consider one habit in our own culture in regard to which there is not this discontinuity of conditioning. With the greatest clarity of purpose and economy of training, we achieve our goal of conditioning everyone to eat three meals a day. The baby's training in regular food periods begins at birth and no crying of the child and no inconvenience to the mother is allowed to interfere. We gauge the child's physiological make-up and at first allow it food oftener than adults, but, because our goal is firmly set and our training consistent, before the child is two years old it has achieved the adult schedule. From the point of view of other cultures this is as startling as the fact of three-year old babies perfectly at home in deep water is to us. Modesty is another sphere in which our child training is consistent and economical; we waste no time in clothing the baby and in contrast to many societies where the child runs naked till it is ceremonially given its skirt or its public sheath at adolescence, the child's training fits it precisely for adult conventions.

In neither of these aspects of behavior is there need for an individual in our culture to embark before puberty, at puberty or at some later date upon a course of action which all his previous training has tabued. He is spared the unsureness inevitable in such a transition.

The illustration I have chosen may appear trivial, but in larger and more important aspects of behavior, our methods are obviously different. Because of the great variety of child training in different families in our society, I might illustrate continuity of conditioning from individual life histories in our culture, but even these, from a comparative point of view, stop far short of consistency and I shall therefore confine myself to describing arrangements in other cultures in which training which with us is idiosyncratic, is accepted and traditional and does not therefore involve the same possibility of conflict. I shall chose childhood rather than infant and nursing situations not because the latter do not vary strikingly in different cultures but because they are nevertheless more circumscribed by the baby's physiological needs than is its later training. Childhood situations provide an excellent field in which to illustrate the range of cultural adjustments which are possible within a universally given, but not so drastic, set of physiological facts.

The major discontinuity in the life cycle is of course that the child who is at one point a son must later be a father. These roles in our society are strongly differentiated; a good son is tractable, and does not assume adult responsibilities; a good father provides for his children and should not allow his authority to be flouted. In addition the child must be sexless so far as his family is concerned, whereas the father's sexual role is primary in the family. The individual in one role must revise his behavior from almost all points of view when he assumes the second role.

I shall select for discussion three such contrasts that occur in our culture between the individual's role as child and as father:

1. responsible—non-responsible status role.
2. dominance—submission,
3. contrasted sexual role.

It is largely upon our cultural commitments to these three contrasts that the discontinuity in the life cycle of an individual in our culture depends.

1. RESPONSIBLE—NON-RESPONSIBLE STATUS ROLE.

The techniques adopted by societies which achieve continuity during the life cycle in this sphere in no way differ from those we employ in our uniform conditioning to three meals a day. They are merely applied to other areas of life. We think of the child as wanting to play and the adult as having to work, but in many societies the mother takes the baby daily in her shawl or carrying net to the garden or to gather roots, and adult labor is seen even in infancy from the pleasant security of its position in close contact with its mother. When the child can run about it accompanies its parents still, doing tasks which are essential and yet suited to its powers, and its dichotomy between work and play is not different from that its parents recognize, namely the distinction between the busy day and the free evening. The tasks it is asked to perform are graded to its powers and its elders wait quietly by, not offering to do the task in the child's place. Everyone who is familiar with such societies has been struck by the contrast with our child training. Dr. Ruth Underhill tells me of sitting with a group of Papago elders in Arizona when the man of the house turned to his little three-year old granddaughter and asked her to close the door. The door was heavy and hard to shut. The child tried, but it did not move. Several times the grandfather repeated, "Yes, close the door." No one jumped to the child's assistance. No one took the responsibility away from her. On the other hand there was no impatience, for after all the child was small. They sat gravely waiting till the child succeeded and her grandfather gravely thanked her. It was assumed that the task would not be asked of her unless she could perform it, and having been asked the responsibility was hers alone just as if she were a grown woman.

The essential point of such child training is that the child is from infancy continuously conditioned to responsible social participation while at the same time the tasks that are expected of it are adapted to its capacity. The contrast with our society is very great. A child does not make any labor contribution to our industrial society except as it competes with an adult; its work is not measured against its own strength and skill but against high-geared industrial requirements. Even when we praise a child's achievement in the home we are outraged if such praise is interpreted as being of the same order as praise of adults. The child is praised because the parent feels well disposed, regardless of whether the task is well done by adult standards, and the child acquires no sensible standard by which to measure its achievement. The gravity of a Cheyenne Indian family ceremoniously making a feast out of the little boy's first snowbird is at the furthest remove from our behavior. At birth the little boy was presented with a toy bow, and from the time he could run about servicable bows suited to his stature were specially made for him by the man of the family. Animals and birds were taught him in a graded series beginning with those most easily taken, and as he brought in his first of each species his family duly made a feast of it, accepting his contribution as gravely as the buffalo his father brought. When he finally killed a buffalo, it was only the final step of his childhood conditioning, not a new adult role with which his childhood experience had been at variance.

The Canadian Ojibwa show clearly what results can be achieved. This tribe gains its livelihood by winter trapping and the small family of father, mother and children live during the long winter alone on their great frozen hunting grounds. The boy accompanies his father and brings in his catch to his sister as his father does to his mother; the girl prepares the meat and skins for him just as his mother does for her husband. By the time the boy is 12, he may have set his own line of traps on a hunting territory of his own and return to his parents' house only once in several months—still bringing the meat and skins to his sister. The young child is taught consistently that it has only itself to rely upon in life, and this is as true in the dealings it will have with the supernatural as in the business of getting a livelihood. This attitude he will accept as a successful adult just as he accepted it as a child.[1]

2. DOMINANCE—SUBMISSION

Dominance—submission is the most striking of those categories of behavior where like does not respond to like but where one type of behavior stimulates the opposite response. It is one of the most prominent ways in which behavior is patterned in our culture. When it obtains between classes, it may be nourished by continuous experience; the difficulty in its use between children and adults lies in the fact that an individual conditioned to one set of behavior in childhood must adopt the opposite as an adult. Its opposite is a pattern of approximately identical reciprocal behavior, and societies which rely upon continuous conditioning characteristically invoke this pattern. In some primitive cultures the very terminology of address between father and son, and more commonly, between grandchild and grandson or uncle and nephew, reflects this attitude. In such kinship terminologies one reciprocal expresses each of these relationships so that son and father, for instance, exchange the same

[1] Landes, Ruth, *The Ojibwa Woman*, Part 1, Youth—Columbia University Contributions to Anthropology, Volume XXXI.

term with one another, just as we exchange the same term with a cousin. The child later will exchange it with his son. "Father—son," therefore, is a continuous relationship he enjoys throughout life. The same continuity, backed up by verbal reciprocity, occurs far oftener in the grandchild-grandson relationship or that of mother's brother-sister's son. When these are "joking" relationships, as they often are, travellers report wonderingly upon the liberties and pretensions of tiny toddlers in their dealings with these family elders. In place of our dogma of respect to elders such societies employ in these cases a reciprocity as nearly identical as may be. The teasing and practical joking the grandfather visits upon his grandchild, the grandchild returns in like coin; he would be led to believe that he failed in propriety if he did not give like for like. If the sister's son has right of access without leave to his mother's brother's possessions, the mother's brother has such rights also to the child's possessions. They share reciprocal privileges and obligations which in our society can develop only between age mates.

From the point of view of our present discussion, such kinship conventions allow the child to put in practice from infancy the same forms of behavior which it will rely upon as an adult; behavior is not polarized into a general requirement of submission for the child and dominance for the adult.

It is clear from the techniques described above by which the child is conditioned to a responsible status role that these depend chiefly upon arousing in the child the desire to share responsibility in adult life. To achieve this little stress is laid upon obedience but much stress upon approval and praise. Punishment is very commonly regarded as quite outside the realm of possibility, and natives in many parts of the world have drawn the conclusion from our usual disciplinary methods that white parents do not love their children. If the child is not required to be submissive however, many occasions for punishment melt away; a variety of situations which call for it do not occur. Many American Indian tribes are especially explicit in rejecting the ideal of a child's submissive or obedient behavior. Prince Maximilian von Wied who visited the Crow Indians over a hundred years ago describes a father's boasting about his young son's intractibility even when it was the father himself who was flouted; "He will be a man," his father said. He would have been baffled at the idea that his child should show behavior which would obviously make him appear a poor creature in the eyes of his fellows if he used it as an adult. Dr. George Devereaux tells me of a special case of such an attitude among the Mohave at the present time. The child's mother was white and protested to its father that he must take action when the child disobeyed and struck him. "But why?" the father said, "he is little. He cannot possibly injure me." He did not know of any dichotomy according to which an adult expects obedience and a child must accord it. If his child had been docile he would simply have judged that it would become a docile adult—an eventuality of which he would not have approved.

Child training which brings about the same result is common also in other areas of life than that of reciprocal kinship obligations between child and adult. There is a tendency in our culture to regard every situation as having in it the seeds of a dominance-submission relationship. Even where dominance-submission is patently irrelevant we read in the dichotomy, assuming that in every situation there must be one person dominating another. On the other hand some cultures, even when the situation calls for leadership do not see it in terms of dominance-submission. To do justice to this attitude it would be necessary to describe their political and especially their economic arrangements, for such an attitude to persist must certainly be supported by economic mechanisms that are congruent with it. But it must also be supported by—or what comes to the same thing, express itself in—child training and familial situations.

3. CONTRASTED SEXUAL ROLE

Continuity of conditioning in training the child to assume responsibility and to behave no more submissively than adults is quite possible in terms of the child's physiological endowment if his participation is suited to his strength. Because of the late development of the child's reproductive organs continuity of conditioning in sex experience presents a difficult problem. So far as their belief that the child is anything but a sexless being is concerned, they are probably more nearly right than we are with an opposite dogma. But the great break is presented by the universally sterile unions before puberty and the presumably fertile ones after maturation. This physiological fact no amount of cultural manipulation can minimize or alter, and societies therefore which stress continuous conditioning most strongly sometimes do not expect children to be interested in sex experience until they have matured physically. This is striking among American Indian tribes like the Dakota; adults observe great privacy in sex acts and in no way stimulate children's sexual activity. There need be no discontinuity, in the sense in which I have used the term, in such a program if the child is taught nothing it does not have to unlearn later. In such cultures adults view children's experimentation as in no way wicked or dangerous but merely as innocuous play which can have no serious consequences. In some societies such play is minimal and the children manifest little interest in it. But the same attitude may be taken by adults in societies where such play is encouraged and forms a major activity among small children. This is true among most of the Melanesian cultures of Southeast New Guinea; adults go as far as to laugh off sexual affairs within the prohibited class if the children are not mature, saying that since they cannot marry there can be no harm done.

It is this physiological fact of the difference between children's sterile unions and adults' presumably fertile sex relations which must be kept in mind in order to understand the different mores which almost always govern sex expression in children and in adults in the same culture. A great many cultures with preadolescent sexual license require marital fidelity and a great many which value premarital virginity in either male or female arrange their marital life with great license. Continuity in sex experience is complicated by factors which it was unnecessary to consider in the problems previously discussed. The essential problem is not whether or not the child's sexuality is consistently exploited—for even where such exploitation is favored in the majority of cases the child must seriously modify his behavior at puberty or at marriage. Continuity in sex expression means rather that the child is taught nothing it must unlearn later. If the cultural emphasis is upon sexual pleasure the child who is continuously conditioned will be encouraged to experiment freely and pleasurably, as among the Marquesans;[2] if emphasis is upon reproduction, as among the Zuni of New Mexico, childish sex proclivities will not be exploited for the only important use which sex is thought to serve in his culture is not yet possible to him. The important contrast with our child training is that although a Zuni child is impressed with the wickedness of premature sex experimentation he does not run the risk as in our culture of associating this wickedness with sex itself rather than with sex at his age. The adult in our culture has often failed to unlearn the wickedness or the dangerousness of sex, a lesson which was impressed upon him strongly in his most formative years.

DISCONTINUITY IN CONDITIONING

Even from this very summary statement of continuous conditioning the economy of such mores is evident. In spite of the obvious advantages, however, there are difficulties in its way. Many primitive societies expect as different behavior from an individual as child and as adult as we do, and such discontinuity involves a presumption of strain.

[2] Ralph Linton, class notes on the Marquesans.

Many societies of this type however minimize strain by the techniques they employ, and some techniques are more successful than others in ensuring the individual's functioning without conflict. It is from this point of view that age-grade societies reveal their fundamental significance. Age-graded cultures characteristically demand different behavior of the individual at different times of his life and persons of a like age-grade are grouped into a society whose activities are all oriented toward the behavior desired at that age. Individuals "graduate" publicly and with honor from one of these groups to another. Where age society members are enjoyed to loyalty and mutual support, and are drawn not only from the local group but from the whole tribe as among the Arapaho, or even from other tribes as among the Wagawaga of Southeast New Guinea, such an institution has many advantages in eliminating conflicts among local groups and fostering intratribal peace. This seems to be also a factor in the tribal military solidarity of the similarly organized Masai of East Africa. The point that is of chief interest for our present discussion however is that by this means an individual who at any time takes on a new set of duties and virtues is supported not only by a solid phalanx of age mates but by the traditional prestige of the organized "secret" society into which he has now graduated. Fortified in this way, individuals in such cultures often swing between remarkable extremes of opposite behavior without apparent psychic threat. For example, the great majority exhibit prideful and nonconflicted behavior at each stage in the life cycle even when a prime of life devoted to passionate and aggressive head hunting must be followed by a later life dedicated to ritual and to mild and peacable civic virtues.[3]

Our chief interest here, however, is in discontinuity which primarily affects the child. In many primitive societies such discontinuity has been fostered not because of economic or political necessity or because such discontinuity provides for a socially valuable division of labor, but because of some conceptual dogma. The most striking of these are the Australian and Papuan cultures where the ceremony of the "Making of Man" flourishes. In such societies it is believed that men and women have opposite and conflicting powers, and male children, who are of undefined status, must be initiated into the male roles. In Central Australia the boy child is of the woman's side and women are tabu in the final adult stages of tribal ritual. The elaborate and protracted initiation ceremonies of the Arunta therefore snatch the boy from the mother, dramatize his gradual repudiation of her. In a final ceremony he is reborn as a man out of the men's ceremonial "baby pouch." The men's ceremonies are

[3] Henry Elkin, manuscript on the Arapaho.

ritual statements of a masculine solidarity, carried out by fondling one another's *churingas*, the material symbol of each man's life, and by letting out over one another blood drawn from their veins. After this warm bond among men has been established through the ceremonies, the boy joins the men in the men's house and participates in tribal rites.[4] The enjoined discontinuity has been tribally bridged.

West of the Fly River in southern New Guinea there is a striking development of this Making of Men cult which involves a childhood period of passive homosexuality. Among the Keraki[5] it is thought that no boy can grow to full stature without playing the role for some years. Men slightly older take the active role, and the older man is a jealous partner. The life cycle of the Keraki Indians includes, therefore, in succession, passive homosexuality, active homosexuality and heterosexuality. The Keraki believe that pregnancy will result from post-pubertal passive homosexuality and see evidences of such practices in any fat man whom even as an old man, they may kill or drive out of the tribe because of their fear. The ceremony that is of interest in connection with the present discussion takes place at the end of the period of passive homosexuality. This ceremony consists in burning out the possibility of pregnancy from the boy by pouring lye down his throat, after which he has no further protection if he gives way to the practice. There is no technique for ending active homosexuality, but this is not explicitly tabu for older men; heterosexuality and children however are highly valued. Unlike the neighboring Marindanim who share their homosexual practices, Keraki husband and wife share the same house and work together in the gardens.

I have chosen illustrations of discontinuous conditioning where it is not too much to say that the cultural institutions furnish adequate support to the individual as he progresses from role to role or interdicts the previous behavior in a summary fashion. The contrast with arrangements in our culture is very striking, and against this background of social arrangements in other cultures the adolescent period of *Sturm und Drang* with which we are so familiar becomes intelligible in terms of our discontinuous cultural institutions and dogmas rather than in terms of physiological necessity. It is even more pertinent to consider these comparative facts in relation to maladjusted persons in our culture who are said to be fixated at one or another pre-adult level. It is clear that if we were to look at our social

[4] Spencer, B., and Gillen, F. J., *The Arunta;* N. Y., Macmillan, 1927 (2 vols.). Róheim, Géza, Psycho-Analysis of Primitive Cultural Types. *Internat. J. Psychoanal.* (1932) 13:1-224—in particular, Chapter III, on the Aranda, The Children of the Desert.

[5] Williams, Francis E., *Papuans of the Trans-Fly;* Oxford, 1936.

arrangements as an outsider, we should infer directly from our family institutions and habits of child training that many individuals would not "put off childish things"; we should have to say that our adult activity demands traits that are interdicted in children, and that far from redoubling efforts to help children bridge this gap, adults in our culture put all the blame on the child when he fails to manifest spontaneously the new behavior or overstepping the mark, manifests it with untoward belligerence. It is not surprising that in such a society many individuals fear to use behavior which has up to that time been under a ban and trust instead, though at great psychic cost, to attitudes that have been exercised with approval during their formative years. Insofar as we invoke a physiological scheme to account for these neurotic adjustments we are led to overlook the possibility of developing social institutions which would lessen the social cost we now pay; instead we elaborate a set of dogmas which prove inapplicable under other social conditions.

"Culture and Personality": A Conceptual Scheme

CLYDE KLUCKHOHN / O. H. MOWRER

Nursing models delineate the basic areas of nursing assessment in terms of biological, psychological, environmental, social, and cultural variables. Each area is further evaluated in relation to patient needs and patient problems. The article by Kluckhohn and Mowrer, although specifically a model for the analysis of personality, adds another dimension to nursing assessment. When the nurse assesses patient behaviors, is she assessing idiosyncratic, role, communal, or universal behaviors? Kluckhohn and Mower's article on culture and personality provides a schema of determinants and levels of abstractions of the determinants in an analysis of personality.

When a nurse works with a single patient, her assessment occurs on the idiosyncratic level, yet a knowledge of the other levels affects her subsequent actions. Nurses interact differently with patients in relation to their biological determinants of sex and age. In addition, nurses anticipate different behaviors from patients according to their classification as male, female, pediatric, adult, or geriatric patients. Nurses have learned that patients will differ in their responses according to their social roles. There is a distinct difference between a nurse or physician who becomes a patient, and a layperson. Patients can

Reproduced by permission of the American Anthropological Association from *The American Anthropologist* 46(1944):1-29.

also be distinguished by the part of the city in which they live, their class or economic group, their value system, their past history, and even the part of the country from which they come. What has been said for idiosyncratic assessment can be said for group assessment as well. The use of this paradigm will add to nursing's knowledge of patients.

"Culture and Personality" is one of the fashionable slogans of contemporary social science and, by present usage, denotes a range of problems which are on the frontier of anthropology and psychology. However, the phrase has unfortunate implications. As Lynd (1939, p. 53) has pointed out, a dualism is implied, whereas "culture *in* personality" and "personality *in* culture" would suggest conceptual models more in accord with our data. Moreover, the slogan favors a dangerous simplification of the problems of personality. A "lust after absolutes," according to John Dewey, is a striking feature of American character structure, and this trend is far from absent in our science. Recognition of culture as one of the determinants of personality is a great gain, but there are some indications that this theoretical advance is tending, in some professional circles, to obscure the significance of the other determinants. Our title, therefore, is a conscious irony. *"Biology and Personality": a Conceptual Scheme* would be equally sensible. Actually, the primary purpose of our article is to show that any consideration of "personality *in* culture" must be carried on within the framework of a complex conceptual scheme which explicitly recognizes instead of tacitly excluding a number of classes of determinants. Just as some investigators have neglected certain determinants, so also have certain investigators remained unaware of the manifold nature of personality and have confused one or two components with the whole personality.

We follow May (1930) in assuming that the parameters of a personality may be defined by a human organism's effects upon others.[1]

[1] We are not unaware of the difficulties into which a rigorous adherence to this definition leads. We see, for example, the implications of Frank's (1935) point: "The conception of the individual 'life space' or 'private world' implies the view that the stimulus-situation, however objectively defined and standardized, will mean to each subject what he projects therein." Our awareness of other problems is indicated in another publication (Mowrer and Kluckholn, 1943). Indeed the position adopted there is appreciably different from that taken here. We feel that this course is justifiable on two grounds. First, in the present confusion in the very difficult terrain of personality theory, we think there is some utility in developing the logical consequences of a widely accepted

All attempts to describe an individual "as he really is" must be regarded as extra-scientific unless they are firmly based upon the regularities in the stimulus value which the individual has *for others.* The only way an observer can "know" other personalities is by noting and making inferences from their social stimulus value—whether in casual social relationships, in controlled interviews, or as manifested in more refined experimental situations such as those provided by the various projective techniques. A subject's own statement of his needs, motives, etc. will normally constitute an important part of the data but can never be taken at their face value without critical evaluation—they must always be interpreted in terms of the reactions of one or more observers. The definition of personality as social stimulus value seems to us one which will permit relatively objective operations.

All scientific theories must take account both of similarities and of differences. A theory of personality must explain equally the ultimate uniqueness of each personality and the observed fact of personality types. More specifically, a conceptual scheme must be adequate to accommodate five generalizations:

1. All human beings have certain properties of social stimulus value, or personality traits, in common. We shall call these *universal* traits, or components, and their antecedents *universal* determinants.
2. The members of any given society tend to share more personality traits with each other than with the members of other societies. We shall call such traits *communal* traits, or components, and their antecedents *communal* determinants.
3. Within a society the behavior characteristic of certain groups or categories of persons shows some constancies. The social stimulus value of those who are playing the same role has a common quality. We shall call this the *role* component and

definition of personality. Second, we are addressing ourselves to two different sets of questions in our two publications. In this article the interest centers upon classificatory abstractions and upon the query: how do we attain our knowledge of personality? The other paper has a point of view which might be designated as "clinical"; the central question is more nearly: what *is* personality? Here personality is seen largely from the standpoint of the reactor; there we try to see personality as it may be imputed to the actor. Perhaps a philosopher might say that the point of view of this paper approaches the "epistemological," that of the other the "ontological." The history of science permits two inductions: 1. it is useful to behave experimentally with respect to conceptual schemes without necessarily claiming "truth" for one to the exclusion of another. 2. a conceptual scheme may be appropriate for analyzing one group of problems, utterly inappropriate for treating the same set of data with a view to a different group of equally legitimate questions.

the antecedents of traits dependent upon roles the *role* determinants.

4. The members of any given society, even those who are playing similar roles, differ among themselves in social stimulus value. We shall call such distinctive and relatively unique traits *idiosyncratic* traits, or components, and their antecedents *idiosyncratic* determinants.
5. Certain similarities, other than those common to all humanity, may be observed in the social stimulus value of individuals from different societies—even where the personality manifestations for those societies vary widely. The possibility of such similarities,is however, deducible from the fact that idiosyncratic determinants are not society-bounded. Consequently, we need no special designation for nor explanation of such similarities.

Our conceptual scheme thus embraces two classes of concepts and their interrelations. On the one hand, there are the *determinants:* those classes of forces which may be abstracted out as influencing social stimulus value. On the other hand, there are the *components* of personality: those facets of the social stimulus value of the individual as an integrate in action which may be regarded as produced primarily by one or another of the classes of determinants.

I: THE DETERMINANTS OF PERSONALITY

First, we must note that this pie, like all others, can be sliced in more than one way. In speaking of the forces operative in personality formation it has been customary to deal with such abstractions as "the biological," "the cultural," "the environmental," and the like. Such abstractive isolates are useful, but, if the primary purpose is to show how total stimulus value may be segregated into various facets or components, these are second-order abstractions. That is, such determining forces as "the biological" and "the cultural" are only elements in abstractions such as "universal" and "communal" which may be linked more immediately to the components of personality. No single component can be regarded as the product of forces which are exclusively biological or cultural. But "the communal component" may be directly connected with the partly biological, partly social, partly cultural, partly physical environmental influences which act upon all members of a single society and which hence may be subsumed as the "communal determinants." Let us now examine systematically and in detail the interdigitation of personality determinants classified as "universal, communal, role, and idiosyncratic" with personality determinants classified in a more familiar manner.

We have heard Clark Hull say "In the beginning there is (a) the organism and (b) the environment." Using this dichotomy as a starting point in analyzing the determinants of personality one might say that the *differences* observed in the personalities of human beings are due to variations in their biological equipment and in the total environment to which they must adjust, while the *similarities* are to be understood as resulting from biological and environmental uniformities. But such an overly general and overly simple formulation—although useful as a first approximation—will not, unless it be further developed, lead us to hypotheses which have predictive value.

We realize, of course, that even the dichotomy which Hull proposes is an abstraction, for, as Henderson (1928) has pointed out, the organism and the environment have a kind of wholeness in the concrete behavioral world which the student loses sight of at his peril. While acknowledging the abstractive nature of the process, it is nevertheless necessary for us to distinguish three aspects of the environment—the physical, the social, and the cultural. Fig. 1 shows in a schematic way how the two classificatory systems cut across each other in a symmetrical manner.

Although the sixteen cells formed by this two-way system of classification are logically exhaustive, the items which are entered in these cells in Fig. 1 are, of course, merely illustrative. The following discussion will expand the significance of each cell, indicate the dynamic interrelatedness of the determinants, give some perspective on present knowledge of each, and further develop the logic of the conceptual scheme as a whole.

Universal, Communal, Role and Idiosyncratic Determinants

The *universal* determinants of personality arise out of four facts: (a) man is an animal of distinctive physical appearance and with somewhat distinctive biological equipment, (b) man is a social animal, (c) man is a cultural animal, (d) man lives in a physical world which obeys natural laws. All human beings normally have two hands and two feet at birth (not four feet and only most exceptionally one hand or three hands). Such properties as stereoscopic vision which differentiate the human species from most other living organisms immediately imply common features of personality. As animals, all men are also bound to face certain problems: they are born; they must breathe, eat, and excrete; they have imperious sexual and other needs; they grow; they face death. As social animals, they must adjust to dependence upon their society and groups within it. As cultural animals, they must adjust to culturally defined expecta-

FIGURE 1—COMPONENTS OF PERSONALITY

Determinants	*Universal*	*Communal*	*Role*	*Idiosyncralic*
Biological	Birth, death, hunger, thirst, elimination, etc.	"Racial" traits, nutrition level, endemic diseases, etc.	Age and sex differences, caste, etc.	Peculiarities of stature, physiognomy, glandular make-up, etc.
Physical-environmental	Gravity, temperature, time, etc.	Climate, topography, natural resources, etc.	Differential access to material goods, etc.	Unique events and "accidents" such as being hit by lightning, etc.
Social	Infant care, group life, etc.	Size, density, and distribution of population, etc.	Cliques, "marginal" men, etc.	Social "accidents" such as death of a parent, being adopted, meeting particular people, etc.
Cultural	Symbolism, tabu on incest and in-group murder, etc.	Traditions, rules of conduct and manners, skills, knowledge, etc.	Culturally differentiated roles	Folklore about accidents and "fate," etc.

*For helpful suggestions as to terminology we are indebted to Drs. Leland H. Jenks, Ralph Linton, and John Whiting. For general discussions which have materially assisted in the clarification of this conceptual scheme we are indebted to Dr. Florence Kluckhohn.

tions. Finally, all men must adapt themselves to an external physical world.

That these facts do constitute problems for human beings is attested by common experience, yet the import and meaning of these facts have not been fully analyzed from the point of view of personality theory, nor do they seem likely to be in the near future for the reason that, being *universal* determinants, their meaning cannot be demonstrated by the usual methods of contrast and comparison. These are background phenomena, the invariables and inevitables to which man must bow and somehow adjust. That "human nature" would be strikingly different from what it is if the human animal had not assumed upright posture and developed prehensile hands, stereoscopic vision, and a nervous system which makes elaborate speech possible goes without saying; and here we have a clearer perception of the significance of this distinctively human cluster of biological traits since we can see what their absence implies in other animals. Contemporary "super-man" fantasies give us perhaps our only glimpse of what human beings would be like if they lived in a world without gravity, temperature, or time.

Since the universal determinants are relatively constant for all mankind, they provide no explanation either of personality typologies or peculiarities. If, however, we notice how certain universal or almost universal experiences (cf. Murray, 1938, p. 287) derive a special phrasing from the interaction of the biological determinants with the realities of the social, cultural, and physical environment, we shall begin our systematic understanding of the observed variation in the social stimulus value of individuals.

All men are born helpless; the external impersonal world presents threats to survival; the human species would disappear completely if social life were abandoned. But the human adaptation to the external world depends not merely upon that mutual support which is social life; it also depends upon culture. Many types of insects live socially yet have no culture. They depend for survival upon behavioral dispositions which are transmitted within the germ plasm. Other organisms show great capacities to learn from experience. Human beings, however, learn not only from experience but also from each other (cf. Linton, 1936, esp. Chaps. V and VI). All human societies rely greatly for their survival upon accumulated learning (culture). All human culture is a storehouse of ready-made solutions to problems which human animals face (Ford, 1939). Into this storehouse are garnered not merely the pooled learning of the men who interact in any one society at any given point in time but also much of the learning of many men long dead, of many men from other societies. This capacity of human beings not only to learn but likewise to teach each other is not the least important of the universal determinants. For example, culture as well as the other three classes of determinants brings it about that throughout the life sequence all men experience both gratifications and deprivations. All persons receive some deprivations and frustrations from the impersonal environment (weather, physical obstacles, and the like interfere with the wishes of men) and from biological conditions (bodily incapacities, illnesses, etc.). Likewise, social life (whether in the ant hill, the beaver colony, the herd, or the human group) means some sacrifice of autonomy, some subordination and superordination. But the pleasure and pain men receive from one another depend not simply on physical facts, biological limitations, and the sheer conditions of social interaction: they depend too upon what the accumulated learning has taught them to expect from one another.

All human personalities are formed under this common condition to demands for conformity to cultural expectation. But the specific character of the cultural expectations varies greatly between different societies and even as between different groups in the same society. This brings us from the universal to the *communal* and *role* determinants. All human beings not only have to be socialized—they are always socialized as members of particular societies and often as members of differentiated categories within the society.

Membership in a society carries with it exposure to determinants of social stimulus value approximately constant for all members of that society. How large or how small a grouping one takes as "a society" is primarily a matter of convenience for the problem in hand. By and large, the physical traits and the total environment of Western Europeans do present a contrast to those of Mohammendans or Eastern Asiatics. White citizens of the United States, in spite of regional, ethnic, and class differences can usually be distinguished, on the basis of their social stimulus value, from Englishmen, Australians, or New Zealanders. From the point of view of personality formation, there is a hierarchy of "societies" to which any individual belongs, ranging from very large units down to the local community.[2] How inclusive a unit one considers in speaking of communal determinants is purely a function of the level of abstraction at which one is operating at a given time.

Some of the personality traits which the members of the same society have in common but which distinguish them from humanity

[2] Cf. Homans (1941, p. 403): "If we return from the word *society* to the facts we had in mind when we used it, we find that these human beings are acting, behaving, that they are acting in response to the actions of one another, and that the interactions are more frequent between fellow members of the society than they are between the 'members' and other men whom we choose to consider outsiders."

as a whole unquestionably derive from distinctive biological heredity. Such persons look alike both to each other and to representatives of other societies. This similarity stems in part from uniformity of clothing and other personal artifacts, but the fact that persons who live together are more likely to be related biologically than are persons who live far apart means that "race" is a biological determinant of personality at the *communal* level of analysis. Biological factors common to a given society may, of course, manifest themselves, not only in terms of appearance, but also, less directly, in behavior. If the metabolic rate is typically low for one group as contrasted with other groups or if certain types of endocrine inbalance are unusually frequent, the social stimulus value of the members of that society will certainly have distinctive qualities. We have as yet, however, very little unequivocal information on this class of determinants (cf. Klineberg, 1935, Chap. VI), but their importance in some cases seems unmistakable.

Likewise, we know almost nothing of what the effects of communal constances in the impersonal environment are upon personality. Does living in continually rainy weather make for different social stimulus value from living in a sunny, arid country? What are the differential effects of living in a walled-in mountain valley, on a flat plain, or upon a high plateau studded with wind-sculptured red buttes? Thus far we can only speculate, for we lack controlled data. The effects of climate (cf. Mills, 1942) and even of topography may be considerable, although they have hardly been rigorously explored.

There are certain social, as opposed to cultural, determinants for each society. Thus the size of the society and the density of the population are certainly not culturally prescribed and are not even altogether determined indirectly by the culture, although often conditioned by the interaction between the technological level of the culture and the exigencies of the physical environment. The location of a population is a determining factor—as well as its size and density. Thus the type of social interaction (with its consequences for personality formation) will be different if a village of 1000 persons occupying an area of one square mile is located in central Kansas or within thirty miles of New York City.

The cultural facet of the environment of any society is a signally important determinant both of the content and of the structure of the personalities of members of that society. The culture very largely determines what is learned: available skills, standards of value, and basic orientations to such universal problems as death. Culture likewise structures the conditions under which learning takes place: whether from parents or parent surrogates or from siblings or from those in the learner's own age grade, whether learning is gradually and gently acquired or suddenly demanded, whether renunciations are harshly enforced or reassuringly rewarded. To say that "culture determines" is, of course, a highly abstract way of speaking. In the behavioral world what we actually see is parents and other older and more experienced persons *teaching* younger and less experienced persons. We assume that biology sets the basic processes which determine *how* man learns, but culture, as the transmitted experiences of preceding generations (both technological and moral) very largely determines *what* man learns (as a member of a society rather than as an individual who has his own private experiences). Culture even determines to a considerable extent how the teaching that is essential to this learning shall be carried out.

Logically, the role determinants could have been encompassed within the communal, for the reference is again to those determinants of personality which operate upon particular groups. But the fact that every society embraces units of social differentiation is so basic and its consequences for personality formation so tremendous (and so often neglected) that the distinction seemed necessary or, at the least, highly useful. In the personality context, the important criterion is always: to what social categories do the individual and those socializing him have a sence of "belongingness" (or of aspiration)? Certain of the categories are fundamentally biological. In every society the organism is differentially socialized according to sex. In every society different behavior is expected of individuals in different age groups,[3] although where these lines are drawn and what behavioral variations are anticipated differs in different cultures. In all known caste societies physical criteria are to some extent involved, and class differentiations are often also tinged with appearance differences. The correlation of the role and physical environmental determinants rests upon the fact that some categories of persons within a society have differential access to residential locations, house types, and material goods generally. As for the role-social determinants, there are always some social groupings (cliques, for example) of enough permanence to be important for personality formation which are neither rationalized along biological lines nor prescribed by the ideal patterns of the culture. Finally, culture regulates the type of behavior deemed appropriate to individuals of a particular age, sex, and status.

That endless *idiosyncratic* variations can and do occur in the life of each human being hardly requires extensive documentation. A child is born a cripple. He is nearly drowned by a sudden flood in a canyon. If the death of a parent means that an infant goes to live with an aged grandmother, or if the remaining parent takes a new mate with a psychopathic personality, the outcome for the child

[3] On the significance of age and sex groups, cf. Linton (1940 and 1942).

must necessarily be different than if the original parent had survived. Even casual social contacts of brief duration ("accidental")—not foreordained by the cultural pattern of social interrelations—often seem crucial in determining whether one's life proceeds along one or another of various possible courses. While some cultures do prescribe different treatment for the oldest or youngest child in a series, the fact that a particular child occupies such a distinctive position is an "accident" from the point of view of the cultural system.

Biological, Physical-Environmental, Social and Cultural Determinants

We have now sketched the manner in which universal, communal, role, and idiosyncratic determinants of personality all include biological, physical, environmental, social, and cultural elements. Let us now reverse the emphasis, taking the classes of determinants along the horizontal axis of Fig. 1 as our point of departure.

There is a vast literature, much of it still highly controversial, on the extent to which biological (organic, constitutional) determinants mold the personality. Here we can scarcely do more than indicate that we recognize the significance of this factor (cf. Woodworth, 1941). At the same time we must also point out the ambiguities of interpretation. As Woodworth (1941, p. 84) observes, "there are serious difficulties in the way of separating the factors of heredity and environment when our interest lies in such traits as human intelligence and personality." Because the individual's body is the one factor which seems to be constant in various situations, some students have succumbed to the temptation of assuming that the biologically inherited idiosyncratic properties of the organism are the chief, if not the sole, determinants of such individual behavioral consistencies. For example, when Jost (1941) reports that the physiological changes produced by frustration vary in different children, it is tempting to jump to the conclusion that these differences represent constitutional differences in frustration tolerance. This may well be an important part of the explanation, but we must not overlook the fact that the children who were studied must necessarily also have had different learning experiences.

Sheldon (1942) submits data purporting to show a high degree of correlation between somatotype and temperament. Newman (1940, p. 172), on the other hand, says that "motor activity and temperament seem to be least influenced by heredity." Rich (1928) obtained correlation coefficients of only 0.20 to 0.30 between metabolism and selected personality traits. Such negative results may, of course, reflect merely the inadequacy of present concepts and research techniques, but certainly the divergent views of contemporary investigators in this field provide little basis for unequivocal conclusions at present. Although there is little doubt that different genetic structures have different potentialities, the complicated interrelations of heredity and environment, which are probably most effectively studied by the methods of co-twin control (see Gesell, 1942), are as yet but little understood. That an interrelation is almost always involved seems to be the best premise for the moment. Therefore, the conclusion of Lynn and Lynn (1938), based on an examination of a large number of subjects, that there is a single organic determinant (face-hand laterality) of "two definite and opposite personality types," must be regarded with reserve, pending independent confirmations.

The old "problem" of "heredity *or* environment" is, then, we feel, essentially meaningless. The only pertinent question is: Which of various genetic potentialities will be actualized as a consequence of a particular series of life-events in a given physical, social, and cultural environment? The particular socialization process institutionalized by a given culture and the accidents peculiar to a given life history may be more or less favorable to the acquisition of certain skills or the development of certain behavior trends, but biology undoubtedly imposes some limitations. There are substantial reasons for believing that learning ability varies greatly on hereditary grounds (Snyder, 1940, pp. 391-399). The various inherited malfunctions are too obvious to require comment. Genetic factors also certainly shape personality through such physical traits as stature, pigmentation, strength, beauty of form, regularity of features, etc. The kind of world one finds about oneself is to a considerable extent determined by the way other people react to one's appearance and physical capacities. Thus, a hunchback does not expect to become a matinee idol, nor a spindle-legged boy a great athlete. Occasionally a physically weak youth, such as Theodore Roosevelt was, may be driven to achieve feats of physical prowess as a kind of over-compensation, but usually the individual accepts exclusion from some types of vocational and social adjustments on the basis of his physical make-up, even though concealed resentments may remain as important ingredients in his total personality. Conversely, special physical fitnesses make certain other types of adjustment particularly cogenial (cf. Cabot, 1938).

Although biology is certainly one of the idiosyncratic determinants of personality, there are only a few extreme cases in which an individual is committed in detail by his particular genetic equipment to particular psychological traits. Even when there is a definite physical handicap, such as deafness (Brunschwig, 1936; Habbe, 1936), the variations are wide. Nevertheless one must always be alive to the possibility of constitutional determinants. Levy (1942) has recently presented evidence for the existence of constitutional factors in maternal behavior. And, as Schilder (1942) says "A constitutional factor would explain why experiences of similar type are in the one case traumatic (producing a point of fixation) and not traumatic in another case." Freeman (1934, pp. 562-570) says, "... one important physiological basis of temperamental differences [is] connected with the reactivity of nervous systems. Various degrees of hyperactivity and hypoactivity of individuals as well as other differences in personality are thought to stem from this fundamental neural difference." This conclusion seems confirmed by the finding of Fries (1937, p. 167) that during the first ten days of life infants vary reliably with respect to amount of activity both during sleep and waking hours, amount of sleep required, sensitivity thresholds, and patterns of response to thwarting. These differences were found to remain "fairly constant" into the third year of life (Fries, 1938, p. 730).

Mendelian genetics have taught us that the particular heredity which a new organism gets from the two genetic lines which are crossing depends upon the accidental way in which the two germ cells exchange chromosomes at the time of fertilization. Except for siblings produced from a single fertilized egg, children having the same parents will have a somewhat different heredity. The idiosyncratic biological determinants which we have been discussing thus take their origin in these "accidents" of the genetic processes. Other idiosyncratic biological determinants exert their forces as a result of some adventitious circumstance during uterine development.

Some factors that we are likely to pigeonhole all too complacently as "biological" often turn out, on careful examination, to be the products of complicated interactions. A crippling illness, for example, may well be partly the consequence of a constitutional predisposition but partly also the consequence of the individual's participation in a caste or class group where sanitation and medical care are inadequate. A tendency toward corpulence certainly has personality implications as well when it is characteristic for a group as when it distinguishes an individual within a group (cf. Bruch, 1941). But the resources of the physical environment as exploited by the culturally available technology are the major determinants of vitamins, noxiants, and nutrition generally, and it is these which have patent consequences for corpulence, stature, and energy potential. If hookworm is endemic in a population, one will hardly expect vigor to be a striking feature of personality (cf. Haldane, 1934, p. 54). Yet hookworm is not an "ineluctable "given," either environmentally or biologically: the effects and prevalence of hookworm are dependent upon culturally enjoined sanitation facilities and other culturally available types of control.

The same complicated sorts of interrelation may be noted between the physical and cultural environments. On the one hand, the physical environment imposes certain limitations upon the cultural forms which man creates or it constrains toward change and re-adjustment in the culture he brings into an ecological area. There is always a portion of the external environment which man can and does adjust to but which he can only very partially control. On the other hand, a part of even the impersonal environment is man-made and cultural. A culture may provide technologies which permit some alternations in the physical world (for example, by irrigation ditches or by terracing of hillsides). There are also those artifacts (houses, furniture, tools, vehicles) which add to the resources for gratification (and frustration). Most important of all, culture screens man's whole perception of the physical world. Sherif (1935) has shown experimentally the effects of social suggestion in setting frames of reference for perception. Hallowell (1935, pp. 20-21) has excellently indicated how culture acts as a set of blinders, or lenses with certain distortions, through which acculturated human beings view the whole world (including other human beings and themselves). Hallowell says:

> Man's psychological responses to the physical objects of his external environment can only be understood... in terms of the traditional meanings which these latter have for him. He never views the outer world freshly or responds to his fellows entirely free from the influences which these meanings exert upon his thought and conduct. Celestial and meteorological phenomena, for example, or the plants and animals of man's habitate, even its inanimate forms, are never separated as such from the concepts of their essential nature and the beliefs about them that appear in the ideological tradition of a particular cultural heritage. Man's attitude toward them is a function of reality as culturally defined, not in terms of their mere physical existence. Thus, to treat the physical environment in which a people lives independently of the meaning that its multiform objects have for that people involves a fundamental psychological distortion if we aim to comprehend the universe which is actually theirs. While useful in certain kinds of analysis, even the assertion that two peoples occupy the same natural environment because the regions inhabited by them exhibit the same climatic type, the same typography and biota can only have significance in the grossest physical sense. It is tantamount to ignoring the very data which have the most important psychological significance, namely the differences in meaning which similar objects of the phenomenal world have for peoples of different cultural traditions. Consequently, the objects of the external world, *as meaningfully defined* in a traditional ideology, constitute the reality to which the individuals habituated to a particular system of

> beliefs actually respond. As applied to the sphere of ecological relations, for example, an inventory of all the natural resources of a specific human habitat does not necessarily correspond to the "natural resources" of that habitat. The physical objects of the environment only enter the reality-order of the human population as a function of specific culture patterns. It is the knowledge and technological level of the culture of a people that determines their natural resources, not the mere presence of physical objects. To people without a tradition of pottery-making the presence of clay in their habitat is no more a natural resource than was the presence of coal and iron in the habitat of the pre-Columbian Indians of eastern North America.

These words, written by an anthropologist, are readily translatable into psychological terms. They say, in effect, that the perceptual, or sign-function, of natural objects (and persons) is greatly influenced by what these objects do to or for man, and they also say that the sign-function of objects is likewise dependent upon what *other persons* say or do in the presence of these objects or their symbolic equivalents. Thus, if a child learns the name of an object and if the child's parents behave in a characteristic manner (e.g., showing fear, approval, or anger) when the child utters the object's name, the child's future reactions to the object itself are certain to be modified. Hence, Hallowell's emphasis upon the importance of knowing how the physical world is *meaningfully defined* if we are to understand its significance and potentialities for a particular person or group of persons.

Just as there are some features of the physical environment that are common to all human beings and just as there are still other features that are relatively distinctive for a given social group, so also are there physical-environmental determinants of personality that are more or less unique for the individual. The fact that no two human beings can occupy the same point at the same time and that the world is never precisely the same on successive occasions means, as many philosophers have pointed out, that, in detail at least, the physical world is idiosyncratic for each individual. That "accidents," such as being burned or perhaps merely frightened by lightning, being struck by a falling tree, or stumbling over an unseen obstacle, have implications for subsequent personality trends can hardly be doubted. More subtle, cumulative influences stemming from the physical environment may also have distinctive consequences for groups or for particular individuals, but these have not been adequately analyzed.

In some ways, the term "impersonal environment" is preferable to "physical environment" because the latter tends to have the exclusive connotation of topography, weather, and the like, whereas actually dwellings, furniture, and all human artifacts are a very important aspect of the external, objective, and non-human environment. These objects all acquire symbolic (including prestige) value for individuals, for social groups, for whole societies. Both symbolically and in the immediate physical sense they are depriving or frustrating agencies. We often speak as if deprivation and frustration were imposed on children only by their elders, but a high shelf which makes a coveted delicacy inaccessible or a gadget which cannot be manipulated will also interfere with a goal response. Societies and social subgroups vary widely in respect to the "material culture" sector of their environments.

The effect of the total environment upon personalities may, following Murray (1938), be called the "press." But, in spite of the subtle interactions of different facets of the environment to which we have been drawing attention, the "press" must be broken down into physical-environmental, social, and cultural. Of these abstractions the most elusive is the social. Although intimately interrelated, the *social* determinants of personality must be distinguished from the cultural. Man is, of course, only one of the many social animals, but the ways in which social, as opposed to solitary, life modifies his behavior are especially numerous and varied. The fact that human beings are mammals and reproduce bi-sexually creates a basic predisposition toward at least the rudiments of social living. And the prolonged helplessness of human infants conduces to the formation of a family group. Although more a product of experience than of any inherent biological force, the in-group principle may also be listed as a universal social determinant. Certain universalistic social processes such as conflict, competition, and accommodation are given their specific forms under the influence of communal social determinants and cultural determinants. Thus, while there is a universal process of social interraction whereby the physically strong tend to dominate the weak, this tendency may be checked and even to some extent reversed by a cultural tradition which rewards intellectual strength more richly than physical strength. Or, the operation of the process may be modified by communal and role social determinants: attitudes toward women, toward infants, toward the old, toward the weak will be conditioned by age and sex ratios and the general population equilibrium prevalent in a given society at a particular time.

Analytically, the distinction between the social and the cultural is a most significant one. This is peculiarly true at the level of the idiosyncratic determinants. There are many forces of social interaction which influence personality formation and yet are in no sense culturally prescribed. As Mead (1930, p. 141) has pointed out, all children (unless multiple births) are born at different points in the parental life careers, which means that they have, psychologically speaking, somewhat different parents. Likewise, whether a child is wanted or unwanted and whether it is of the desired sex will also determine the specific ways in which its parents and other will treat it—even though the culture says that all children are wanted and defines the two sexes as of equal value.

In the concrete, however, the social and cultural are, for the most part, almost inextricably mixed. Let us take as an example a case where "accidents" of the life history are superimposed (as idiosyncratic determinants) upon both biological and cultural determinants. Even though identical twins may differ remarkably little from a constitutional standpoint and may also have culturally defined experiences which are very similar, unpredictable factors in the impersonal environment may impinge upon them so that their social interactions are quite different. If, for instance, one of two such twins happened to be injured in an automobile accident and the other was not, and if the injured twin has to spend a year in bed, it is plausible to suppose that marked personality differences might result.[4] But the variations in the social treatment which the bed-ridden twin receives will be partly determined by culture (the extent to which the ideal patterns say that a sick child must be petted etc.), partly by extra-cultural factors: the mother's need for nurturance, the father's idiomatic variant of his culturally patterned role in these circumstances, etc.

"Culture," though definitely an abstraction (cf. Kluckhohn, 1941, p. 126), is, like "heredity," a highly convenient conceptual construct. Indeed, culture is precisely one form of heredity—social as opposed to biological heredity (cf. Linton, 1936, pp. 77-79, and 85). Thus, just as we may speak of "constitutional determinants of personality," so equally are we justified in speaking of "cultural determinants of personality." This is not resorting to mysticism or to an abstraction which is not reducible to its behavioral referents. Nothing is more certain and concrete than the fact of human teaching. An example will, however, show the justification for detaching the teaching itself from the actual teachers. If a random third of the parents of Cambridge, Massachusetts, were to die tomorrow and their children were to be socialized by their surviving relatives and friends in Cambridge, it may safely be predicted that what these children would learn would be approximately the same—taking the group as a statistical whole—as if their parents had survived. In other words, although culture is always mediated by individuals—and this fact must *never* be forgotten—it does, in a limited sense, have a supra-individual character. The existence and con-

[4]The extent to which these differences persisted into adulthood would, to be sure, depend upon many factors, but it is unlikely that they would be counteracted entirely.

tinuity of most of any culture does not depend upon the lives of any *particular* person or persons in that group. Indeed, in moderately stable societies, although the whole population of any one period will, over a period of years, die, the culture will have been transmitted to their descendants and will continue in existence with a modicum of change. One may compare with this the fact that the genes of persons now long dead continue to exert their effects upon the behavior of living descendants.

Anthropology has made what is perhaps its most distinctive contribution by calling attention to the sparsity of *universal* cultural determinants of personality. It has shown that many social values which were formerly assumed to be common to all humanity are functions of a particular culture. But the cross-cultural analyses of the anthropologists have left a few universals. All societies have tabus on incest. All societies teach that it is "wrong" to murder members of one's own social group. And all societies have as part of their culture the precept of loyalty to the in-group.

In order for culture, in the sense of accumulated and transmitted discoveries and skills, to be maximally effective and useful to succeeding generations, its content must have a certain generality and common applicability. That most of the cultural determinants are of the communal and role types is obvious. Yet, in a sense, certain cultural determinants are idiosyncratic in their reference. In small societies, for example, there may well be but a single dwarf. One culture prescribes that a dwarf shall be laughed at, another that he be regarded with reverence as a supernatural being. Here again we must note the interdependence of the determinants. The effects of "accidents" upon the individual and upon the behavior of others toward him are influenced by culture and indeed by all the communal and role determinants. No society entirely fails to try to prepare individuals for the uncertainties as well as for the culturally predictable "certainties" of life. Most cultures contain preconceptions about the import of "accidents" and "misfortunes." It is, for example, definitely a part of the traditional lore of some societies that disapproved conduct will be punished by "fate" in one way or another.[5] Illness, untimely death, famine, deformity, defeat in war, floods, and other natural catastrophes are interpreted as causally related to previous action on the part of individuals or the group as a whole (Hallowell, 1941; Kluckhohn, 1942). In other societies culture may not prescribe that misfortune shall follow socially objectionable behavior, but when misfortunes do occur, such causes may be looked for retrospectively. Still other

[5] For an illuminating discussion of the relation between the concept of fate and parental influences, see Fenichel (1934).

instances might be cited in which culture provides magical interpretations of uncontrollable events; and each culture must, by virtue of slight uncontrollable and unpredictable deviations in what and how and by whom the individual person is socialized, have for the individual slightly private versions and overtones. But by its very nature culture must be less concerned with the variable than with the relatively constant experiences which human beings encounter, although, as we have seen, it is not entirely meaningless to speak of *idiosyncratic* cultural determinants of personality.

Constants and Variables

While the significance of biological determinants has been, and in popular circles still is, over-estimated, there are some indications that social scientists are tending to give the same misguided unilateral evaluation to culture. The problem must never be structured as biological *or* cultural determinants. The prime point in the foregoing discussion is that physical-environmental, social, cultural, and biological determinants and their complicated interrelations must *all* be given due consideration.

Finally, it must be continually realized that, from the point of view of the vertical columns in Fig. 1, some classes of determinants may be regarded as "constants," others as "variables." The idiosyncratic determinants can be called "variables" in contrast to the other three classes which, with fair precision, may be termed "constants" (either for all men or for social units of men—nations, communities, castes, classes, etc.). Because of personality typologies and folkloristic social stereotypes the constants are not likely to be forgotten. But we sometimes overlook the forces operative in personality formation which cannot be predicted upon the basis of knowledge of a biological stock, a physical environment, the general properties of social interaction, and a given culture. They are the thing that "just happen to people"—private to the individual rather than more or less inevitable for all individuals who have a common heredity, share a physical environment, live in a society of a certain size and having other non-cultural determinants of social interaction, and share a common culture. The potentialities for such happenings are obviously present in the system as defined by the communal and role determinants, but they are not prescribed by the total system for all individuals of a certain age, sex, class, or other social category.

Individuals not only have biological and social experiences, but they have experiences which could not have been predicted from the nature of the human body or from membership in a specific society. Putting the conceptual scheme in a manner which cuts across both the constants and the variables we have (a) the organism moving through a field which is (b) structured both by culture and by the physical and social world in a relatively uniform manner but which is (c) subject to endless variation within the general patterning, due to special, or idiosyncratic determinants which are introduced by "accident," or "fate."[6]

II: THE COMPONENTS OF PERSONALITY

> There are fashions in personality. Fashions that vary in time—like crinolines and hobble skirts—and fashions that vary in space—like Gold Coast loin-cloths and Lombard Street tail-coats. In primitive societies everyone wears, and longs to wear, the same personality. But each society has a different psychological costume. Among the red Indians of the Northwest Pacific Coast the ideal personality was that of a mildly crazy egotist competing with his rivals on the plane of wealth and conspicuous consumption. Among the Plains Indians, it was that of an egotist competing with others in the sphere of war-like exploits. Among the Pueblo Indians, the ideal personality was neither that of an egotist, nor of a conspicuous consumer, nor of a fighter, but of the perfectly gregarious man who makes great efforts never to distinguish himself, who knows the traditional rites and gestures and tries to be exactly like everyone else.
>
> European societies are large and racially, economically, professionally heterogeneous; therefore orthodoxy is hard to impose, and there are several contemporaneous ideals of personality. (Note that Fascists and Communists are trying to create one single "right" ideal—in other words are trying to make industralized Europeans behave as though they were Dyaks or Eskimos. The attempt, in the long run, is doomed to failure; but in the meantime, what fun they will get from bullying the heretics!)
>
> In our world, what are the ruling fashions? There are, of course, the ordinary clerical and commercial modes—turned out by the little dressmakers round the corner. And then *La haute couture. Ravissante personalité d'intérieur de chez Proust. Maison Nietzsche et Kipling: personalité de sport. Personalité de nuit, création de Lawrence. Personalité de bain, par Joyce.* . . . A pragmatist would have to say that Ben Jonson's psychology was "truer" than Shakespeare's. Most of his contemporaries did in fact perceive themselves and were perceived as Humours. It

[6] Cf. Young (1941, pp. 132-136) and Kluckhohn (1939, especially footnote 6).

took Shakespeare to see what a lot there was outside the boundaries of the Humour, behind the conventional mask. But Shakespeare was in a minority of one—or, if you set Montaigne beside him, of two. Humours "worked"; the complex, partially atomized personalities of Shakespeare didn't.

In the story of the emperor's new clothes, the child perceives that the great man is naked. Shakespeare reversed the process. His contemporaries thought they were just naked Humours; he saw that they were covered with a whole wardrobe of psychological fancy dress.

Take Hamlet, Hamlet inhabited a world whose best psychologist was Polonius. If he had known as little as Polonius, he would have been happy. But he knew too much; and in this consists his tragedy. Read his parable of the musical instruments. Polonius and the others assumed as axiomatic that man was a penny whistle with only half a dozen stops. Hamlet knew that potentially at least, he was a whole symphony orchestra.

Mad Ophelia lets the cat out of the bag. "We know what we are, but we know not what we may be." Polonius knows very clearly what he and other people *are*, within the ruling conventions. Hamlet knows this, but also what they may be—outside the local system of masks and humours.

To be the only man of one's age to know what people may be as well as what they conventionally are! Shakespeare must have gone through some rather disquieting quarters of an hour.

—Aldous Huxley (*Eyeless in Gaza*, pp. 105-107)

Although in the literary rather than in the scientific mode, Huxley is here calling attention to certain very real problems in personality theory. If the purpose of the first section was to avoid the pitfalls of an over-simple delineation of the determinants of the social stimulus value of individuals, the purpose of this section is to stress the necessity of treating the individual as an integrate in action. One must not confuse certain limited aspects of social stimulus value with the whole personality. In certain circumstances, we react to men and women, not as unique organizations of experience, but as representatives of a group. In other circumstances, we react to them primarily as fulfilling certain roles. But if at times certain facets draw our attention more than others, we must not lose sight of the fact that the personality, like the organism whose social stimulus value it represents, is a whole. Often the best way to avoid confusing a part with a whole is to become explicitly aware of the specific parts which may be abstracted from the whole. Let us therefore follow out in some detail the implications of the varying "psychological costumes" of different societies in space and in time and of the "Humours."

The Universal Component

In our preoccupation with the interesting differences which we note between individuals and personality types, we tend to forget that the phrase, "a common humanity," is not altogether meaningless. The reaction which any human being produces in other human beings is different from that produced by any other kind of animal or by any sort of inanimate entity or event. The folkloristic saying, "Why, that isn't even *human,*" is based, as are so many commonplaces, upon a frequently overlooked but profound truth: the basic uniformities in physical appearance and behavior deeply condition the social stimulus value of all men for all other men. These stem from the universal (biological, physical-environmental, social, and cultural) determinants which have been reviewed in the preceding section and constitute what we may designate as the *universal component* in the personality of all human beings. By using the expression, "all human beings," we tend to exclude from this generalization those individuals who, because of idiocy, physical monstrosity, or social isolation and neglect, fail to qualify for responsible membership in their natural social group. Properly speaking, the universal component of human personality consists of those physical and behavioral traits which are accepted as normal and desirable in *all* human societies. The facts of personality which compose this universal component have been the subject of much speculation, but we have little scientifically verified information concerning them. We mention the universal component of personality in the present context, partly for purposes of conceptual completeness and partly as a means of indicating important lacunae in our knowledge.

The Communal Component

That "the members of any given society tend to share more personality traits with other members of that society than with the members of other societies" is attested by common experience. If we are unfamiliar with Navaho Indians, we are likely to react to them first as Navahos rather than as individuals. Their first social stimulus value is largely in terms of those features of physical appearance, costume, and behavior which sets them off as representatives of a different society from our own. One frequently hears whites who have recently entered the Navaho country say, "I can't tell one Indian from another." Similarly, one hears Navahos who have had little experience with whites saying, "All white women seem alike to me. I just can't recognize one after I have met her."

This diffuse generalization of the social stimulus value of members of a particular out-group certainly rests, in the first instance, upon similarities of total visual (and sometimes olfactory) impression. Such also seems to be the basis of that rather remarkable phenomenon: species cohesion in animals (cf. Zuckerman, 1933, pp. 115-118). With human beings, however the failure to make strictly individual discriminations goes immediately from physical appearance on to behavior, first of all linguistic behavior. Even within a larger social unit the reactor places the actor as the representative of a regional or class group on the basis of "accent." To a considerable degree, physical appearance and accent are reacted to only as symbols of a more thorough-going and deeply felt differentiation. What "sets off" our reaction in the first instance may be a combination of physical traits—but skin color, nose shape, and other physical features are in certain cases closely associated with our experience of certain culturally determined varieties of behavior.

The tendecny towards uniformity in social stimulus value may be observed even as between social groups where differences in physique and distinctive costume are slight and inconstant (for example, between Englishmen or Australians and Americans). In this case also, the first contacts with representatives of the alien society are likely to have more the character of culture-defining value than of person-defining value (cf. Sapir, 1934, p. 409). The statistical prediction can safely be made that one hundred Americans will display particular features of personal organization and behavior more frequently than will a hundred Englishmen of comparable age, social class, and vocational assortment. So great is the influence of culture that there is a grain of truth in Faris' (1934, p. 7) statement that "Culture is the collective side of personality; personality the subjective aspect of culture." But this is rather less than a half-truth. Not only culture but also the other communal determinants—the common forces in the biological heredity and the physical and social environments—bring about that configuration of personality traits which the members of a given society tend to share. Since any organism is a whole and since in the last analysis the social stimulus value of the organism is a totality, we shall not call those *aspects* of social stimulus value which accrue to the individual as a member of a society the "communal personality" but rather the *communal component*[7] of personality.

[7] In speaking of "the communal component of personality" we are getting at something quite similar to, though more inclusive than, Kardiner's (1939) "basic personality structure." The adjective "basic" seems to us unfortunate and misleading. For idiosyncratic determinants do not enter into the formation of the "basic personality structure" and yet they are actually more "basic" in the sense that many of the biological idiosyncratic determinants exist prior to all cultural training. Moreover, if an Englishman came to this country when he was five and remained here, he would certainly acquire most of the American

The Role Component

But we must deal with "Humours" as well as with "psychological costumes." Still another closely related abstraction must be added if we are not to be misled by certain relatively surface resemblances between personalities. Under the influence of the role determinants the communal component takes many variant forms. It is an induction from common experience that Englishmen occupying different statuses have different social stimulus value for the same persons. The peer's personality is not that of the cab driver nor that of the retired Indian colonel. The personalities of American women tend to be distinguished by certain traits which appear much less frequently in the personalities of American men. When we meet new people at a social gathering, we are often able to predict correctly, "That man is a doctor." "That man certainly isn't a business man—he acts like a professor." "He surely isn't an artist or a writer or an actor."

There is nothing mysterious about all this. As Linton (1936, pp. 476-477) says:

> Each society approves and rewards certain combinations of qualities when they appear in individuals occupying particular statuses. Furthermore, it tries to develop these qualities in all the individuals for whom the particular statuses can be forecast. In other words, each society has a series of ideal personalities which correspond to the various statuses which it recognizes. Such status personalities are not to be confused with with psychological types. In their definition societies do not go far below the surface. The status personality does not correspond to the total personality but simply to certain aspects of the content and more superficial orientations of the latter, i.e., to those elements of the total personality which are immediately concerned with the successful performance of the individual's roles.

These considerations explain the observed fact that the account of an individual's personality which we get from equally competent observers who have known him when he was carrying out different roles—in the home, in business, in the clinic, in his lodge—often fail to coincide in important particulars. Few individuals are "single, consistent personalities." Most individuals have "different faces" to put on for each situation that arises. There are not only, as John Dewey says, "occupational psychoses"—there are also "occupational

"communal component" which would be superimposed (i.e., "based") upon the structure arising out of constitution and his earlier socialization in England. However, Kardiner really means "basic" in the sense of "uniform" or "common to members of a group," and his conception is therefore closely related to ours.

personalities" (cf. Hughes, 1928, 1937)—which is perhaps but a slightly different way of saying the same thing. Merton (1940) writes of "bureaucratic personality structure." Landes (1937) even talks of the "summer and winter personalities" of the Ojibway Indians. Other writers speak of "age and sex personalities," having in mind such phenomena as the following: the personality of an old doctor is different from that of a young one; the personality of the woman lawyer has typical differences from that of her male colleague.

The differential aspects of personality manifestations which are reacted to and observed when the individual carries out the differing roles of his social life we shall call the *role component.* We shall not speak of the "role personality," for this implies that the personality is divisible, whereas it is a whole, separable only by abstraction. If the terms we use for our abstractions do not imply absolute divisibility but merely facets to which we may differentially react, we are less likely to forget that, when we speak of "personality," we are always necessarily referring to the individual as an integrate in action. The fact that a doctor has a bedside manner does not mean that he ceases to act as an American or in accord with the idiosyncratic core of his personality. We use the term "role" rather than "status" because the distinction which Davis (1942, p. 310) makes between "status" and "office" is a useful one and because, as Davis (p. 311) also points out, the social stimulus value of the individual carrying out a role "is always influenced by factors other than the stipulations of the position itself."

The relative weight of the role component in the social stimulus value of any person varies greatly according to the number of roles defined and the accent of the expectations enjoined by different cultures. Fromm's (1941) observations are acute:

> A person [in medieval society] was identical with his role in society; he was a peasant, an artisan, a knight, and not *an individual* who *happened* to have this or that occupation... The "self" in the interests of which modern man acts is the *social* self, a self which is essentially constituted by the role the individual is supposed to play and which in reality is merely the subjective disguise for the objective social function of man in society.... The pseudo self is only an agent who actually represents the role a person is supposed to play but who does so under the name of the self. It is true that a person can play many roles and subjectively be convinced that he is "he" in each role. Actually he is in all these roles what he believes he is expected to be, and for many people, if not most, the original self is completely suffocated by the pseudo self.... When

the general plot of the play is handed out, each actor can act vigorously the role he is assigned and even make up his lines and certain details of the action by himself. Yet he is only playing a role that has been handed over to him." (pp. 41-42, 117, 205, 253).

The Idiosyncratic Component

Alexander (1942, p. 244) remarks that a persistent organization of trends and tendencies of the individual is formed early in life "by combination of hereditary and domestic influences." He partially recognizes what we should call the "communal component" when he says, "These domestic influences differ enough from family to family to produce a wide variety of personality structures which might be rare in one civilization but common in another." But he correctly points out that only some of the "domestic influences" are "typical of contemporary society rather than peculiar to the individuals, whether parents or siblings, who exercise them." And Alexander is probably right in saying, "The individuality of parents has a greater influence upon the development of their children's personalities than convention and cultural tradition" (p. 243).

Biological, cultural, social, and physical environmental determinants all combine to produce the *idiosyncratic component* of personality. Smith is "stubborn" in his office as well as in his home and in a golf game. He would have been "stubborn" in all social contexts if he had been taken to England from America at an early age and his socialization had been completed there. The idiosyncratic component always tinges the playing of roles. The social stimulus value of different individuals in the same society who occupy the same position (statuses and offices) varies. We verbalize such differences by saying, "Yes, Smith and Jones are both forty-five year old Americans, both small business men with about the same responsibilities and prestige—but somehow they are different." Each individual's patterned ways of perceiving, feeling, and behaving do have a characteristic organization which is not precisely paralleled by that of any other individual. For purposes of therapy and for certain research objectives, it is this uniqueness of personality which must be tenaciously accented. But for general scientific purposes both facts must be kept firmly in mind: the uniqueness of personalities and their resemblances. The idiosyncratic features are, as it were, imbedded in a matrix which is more public than private, and only the totality—not any one component—may properly be called the personality. Even though we live in a society where "who you are rather than what you are counts," the role component is only one face of the self. On the other hand, the idiosyncratic component, like the communal and role components, is equally only one part of the individual's total social stimulus value. When Davis and Dollard (1940, p. 11) speak of personality as "that behavior of an individual which distinguishes him from other individuals *trained by similar social controls*," they do violence to the intricate interdependence of the three components.

In the preceding section we called attention to the fact that in addition to universal and communal resemblances in the personalities of different human beings, there is another type of resemblance which cuts across the boundaries of groups but which is due to idiosyncratic rather than to universal determinants. This observation can be concretely illustrated. In general, Hopi Indians and white Americans have very different social stimulus value. But occasionally one meets a Hopi whose behavior, either by total impression or by some single reaction system, reminds one very strongly of the behavior of certain white men or women. Such parallels could orginate from a similarity either in biological, physical-environmental, social or cultural idiosyncratic determinants. A Hopi and a white man could both have a special endocrine imbalance unusual in the populations of both societies. Or both Hopi and white could have had long childhood illnesses which brought them each an exceptional amount of maternal devotion. While the effects of extra maternal care would have somewhat different effects according to the prevailing constellation of the other determinants, there would remain at least a segmental similarity which might well produce arresting resemblances in the two adult personality structures.

Discrimination of the Components: Actors and Reactors

It is not unenlightening to remember that in early Latin *persona* means "a mask"—*dramatis persona* is thus an actor who wears a mask in a play (cf. Mauss, 1938, Horney, 1939, esp. Chap. XIII). Etymologically and historically, then, a personality is the wearer of a mask. For those who are fairly well adjusted in their society, the communal and role components of the personality do tend to constitute disguises. Just as the outer body screens the viscera from view and clothing the genitals, so the "public" facets of personality shield the private personality from the curious and conformity-demanding world of other persons—and usually, also, keep many motivations from the individual's own consciousness. The person who has painfully achieved some sort of integration and who knows what is expected of him in a particular social situation will produce those responses with only a slight indiosyncratic coloring. This is why the uniformities provided by the communal and role components can, in the case of "normal" individuals, be penetrated only by the long-continued, intensive, and oblique procedures of depth psychology. Only projective techniques will often bring out what the individual does not want to tell about himself and what he himself often does not know.

Some of our analogies perhaps suggest that any personality may be dissected as one peels the layers off an onion. This is a crude and only very partially correct view. Sometimes the communal component is the outer "layer," sometimes the role component. This depends upon who the observer is. For social stimulus value is a function both of actor and of reactor. If the actor is from a society markedly different from that of the observer, his social stimulus value is at first almost completely confused with the communal component. What are actual peculiarities of the individual may be atrributed to a stereotype for that society. The role component is hardly perceived at all unless the reactor is familiar with social differentiations in the other society. Roles can be discriminated with refinement only if the "audience" can appreciate differences. The delicacy of "identification" or "placement" depends on this. Thus we see why evaluations of out-groupers as individuals are always more or less inaccurate. Here we have one important aspect of "race prejudice"—individuals are judged on the basis of stereotypes. Discriminations are not sensitive. The kind of person one is taken to be is determined entirely by the kind of people that one habitually has around one.

When one first meets a new person in one's own society, particularly if the person be from an occupational group sharply different from one's own or if the situation be an unfamiliar one, the stimulus value of the person is likely to derive primarily from the role component. If, however, one wants really to comprehend the total personality, one must "get behind" this front, temporarily stripping off (but not forgetting) the outer layer which is the totality of responses expected of the individual (for example, as young man, as lawyer, as lawyer dealing with female client, etc.). Before the student can get to the idiosyncratic component he must also "factor out" the communal component. Apart from the fact that the subject is thirty years old, a man, and a lawyer, he is also an American. Many personality traits he will also share with American men, with American old people, with barbers and factory workers.

Making the distinctions between *universal*, *communal*, *role*, and *idiosyncratic* components is not a mere exercise in sterile taxonomy. Clarity and consistency in these discriminations is essential to sound work in the "culture and personality" field. Otherwise we shall continually run the danger of ascribing to some known "accident" of the individual's life history, a trait which he actually shares with almost all other Americans who have not been subjected to that event-process at all. Or we shall interpret a person's behavior in a given situation as reflecting certain trends in his "core personality" (idiosyncratic component) when he is only conforming, very acceptably, to social expectations of performance of that role. Only after careful scrutiny can behavior be taken at its face value as providing clues to the idiosyncratic variant of socially approved norms which any human organism's action represents. All of us, even clinicians, are sometimes "taken in" by the masks of the communal and role components. We visit a doctor in his office, and his behavior conforms so perfectly to our expectations that we say, often mistakenly, "There is indeed a well-adjusted personality." We extrapolate from his behavior in his role of physician and infer, "There is a respectable citizen if there ever was one. Obviously his private life also conforms to prevalent standards."

The reader may have wondered why we have designated four personality components corresponding, respectively, to the universal, communal, role, and idiosyncratic determinants of personality but have not equally discriminated components which correspond to the biological, physical-environmental, social and cultural determinants. As we have already indicated, the latter seem to us to represent higher order abstractions than do the universal, communal, role, and idiosyncratic determinants; and common experience shows that there are no personality components, or traits, stemming from these second-order determinants which are so easily discerned as are those which derive from the first-order determinants. This is because, in all save new-born organisms, the biological and environmental aspects of personality manifestations can hardly be disentangled. All geneticists are agreed today that "traits" are not inherited in any simple sense: observed characters of growing and matured organisms are, at any given point in time, the product of complex interactions between biologically inherited potentialities or trends and environmental influences. On the other hand, it *is* possible by simple observation and induction to determine the features of personality shared by the members of a given society, by those playing a common role, etc. Freud, Murray (1938), and other clinical writers have proposed personality sub-divisions which are suggestive of our four second-order determinants. This, however, is a complicated problem which cannot be adequately discussed here but has been considered in some detail elsewhere (Mowrer and Kluckhohn, 1943).

SUMMARY

Starting with May's definition of personality as an individual's "social stimulus value," we have sought to delineate a conceptual scheme which would accommodate all of the *determinants* of social stimulus value and which would also systematically order the *components* of "personality" as thus defined. A survey of the evidence indicates that the determinants of personality fall naturally into four categories: *universal* determinants, *communal* determinants, *role* determinants, and *idiosyncratic* determinants. Further analysis shows that these categories, which may be represented as the headings of four vertical columns (Fig. 1), are cut across horizontally by another four-fold classification of determinants which includes: *biological* determinants, *physical-environmental* determinants, *social* determinants, and *cultural* determinants. There thus emerges an exhaustive matrix of sixteen sub-categories, or "cells," to one of which any naturalistic determinant of personality can be logically assigned.

When the four vertical, or first-order, determinants of personality are examined, it is found that they rather exactly parallel four components, or "layers," of personality which are tacitly assumed, if not explicitly distinguished, by contemporary social science, namely, the *universal* component, the *communal* component, the *role* component, and the *idiosyncratic* component. Personality components which similarly correspond to the horizontal, or second-order, determinants of personality are less readily identified, although the "mental anatomy" of psychoanalysis, with its *id*, *ego*, and *super-ego* categories, may be said to parallel in a very rough way the *biological*, *physical-environmental*, *social*, and *cultural* categories of personality determinants.

We should like to stress our position that we do not in any sense claim an absolute superiority for our terminology. We acknowledge, for example, the utility of the *id*, *ego*, and *super-ego* divisions within the psychoanalytic frame of reference. We are aware of the difficulties of the "social stimulus value" definition of personality, although we strongly disagree that this definition implies than an individual has "two personalities" because his effects upon two observers are markedly different. Rather, we insist, this datum indicates only that the actor-reaction equation must be considered in all personality studies. Thus, when a person does produce divergent effects upon two reactors, this almost always reflects varying facets in the personal organization of *both* actor and reactor. We do suggest that our conceptual scheme is in accord with many recent studies in this field. Our "communal personality," for instance, is very similar to Fromm's (1941, p. 277) "social character."

Finally, our realization that all of the personality determinants and all of the personality components are abstractions must be emphasized again. Concretely, we can only follow the whole organism as an integrate in action (cf. Frank, 1935).

BIBLIOGRAPHY

Alexander, F. 1942. Our age of unreason. New York: Lippincott and and Co.

Boas, F. 1938. The mind of primitive man. (2d ed.) New York: Macmillan and Co.

Bruch, H. 1941. Obesity in childhood and personality development. American Journal of Orthopsychiatry, 11, 467-475.

Brunschwig, L. 1936. A study of some personality aspects of deaf children. New York: Teachers College, Columbia University.

Cabot, P. S. de Q. 1938. The relationship between characteristics of personality and physique in adolescents. Genetic Psychological Monograph, 20, 3-120.

Davis, A. and J. Dollard. 1940. Children of bondage. Washington, D. C.: American Council on Education.

Davis, K. 1942. A conceptual analysis of stratification. American Sociological Review, 7, 309-322.

Faris, E. 1934. Culture and personality among the forest Bantu. Publication of the American Sociological Society, vol. 28.

Fenichel, O. 1934. Outline of clinical psychoanalysis. New York: W. W. Norton and Co.

Ford, C. S. 1939. Society, culture, and the human organism. The Journal of General Psychology, 20, 135-179.

Frank, L. K. 1935. Structure, function, and growth. Philosophy of Science, 2, 210-236.

Freeman, G. L. 1934. Introduction to physiological psychology. New York: Ronald Press Co.

Fries, M. 1937. Factors in character development, neuroses, psychoses and delinquency. American Journal of Orthopsychiatry, 7, 142-182.

_____. 1938. Interrelated factors in development. American Journal of Orthopsychiatry, 8, 726-753.

Fromm, E. 1941. Escape from freedom. New York: Farrar and Rinehart.

Gesell, A. 1942. The method of co-twin control. Science, 95, 446-449.

Habbe, S. 1936. Personality adjustments of adolescent boys with impaired hearing. New York: Teachers College, Columbia University.

Haldane, J. B. S. 1934. Anthropology and human biology. In Compte-rendu, Congres International des Sciences Anthropologiques et Ethnologiques, 53-65.

Hallowell, A. I. 1935. Handbook of psychological leads for ethnological field workers, Mimeographed.

_____. 1941. The social function of anxiety in a primitive society. American Sociological Review, 6, 869-882.

Henderson, L. J. 1928. Blood, a study in general physiology. New Haven: Yale University Press.

Homans, G. C. 1941. English villagers of the thirteenth century. Cambridge, Mass.: Harvard University Press.

Horney, K. 1939. New ways in psychoanalysis. New York: W. W. Norton and Co.

Hughes, E. C. 1928. Personality types and the division of labor. American Journal of Sociology 33, 754-768.

_____. 1937. Institutional office and the person. American Journal of Sociology, 43, 404-414.

Jost. H. 1941. Some psychological changes during frustration. Child Development, 12, 9-15.

Kardiner, A. 1939. The Individual and his society. New York: Columbia University Press.

Klineberg, O. 1935. Race differences. New York: Harper and Brothers.

Kluckhohn, C. 1939. Theoretical bases for an empirical method of studying the acquisition of culture by individuals. Man, 39. No. 89.

_____. 1941. Patterning as exemplified in Navaho culture. In Spier, L., ed., Language, culture, and personality. Menasha, Wis.: Sapir Memorial Publication Fund.

_____. 1942. Myths and rituals: a general theory. Harvard Theological Review, 35, 45-80.

Landes, R. 1937. The personality of the Ojibwa. Culture and Personality, 6, 51-60.

Levy, D. 1942. Psychosomatic aspects of some aspects of maternal behavior. Psychosomatic Medicine, 4, 223-228.

Linton, R. 1936. The study of man. New York: Century Co.

_____. 1940. A neglected aspect of social organization. American Journal of Sociology, 45, 870-887.

_____. 1942. Age and sex categories. American Sociological Review, 7, 589-604.

Lynd, R. 1939. Knowledge for what? Princeton: Princeton University Press.

Lynn, J. G. and D. R. Lynn 1938. Face-hand laterality in relation to personality. Journal of Abnormal and Social psychology, 33, 291-323.

Mauss, M. 1938. Une categorie de l'esprit humain: la notion de Personne, celle de moi. Journal of the Royal Anthropological Institute, 68, 263-283.

May, M. A. 1930. A comprehensive plan for measuring personality. In Proceedings and Papers of the Ninth International Congress of Psychology, pp. 298-300. Princeton, New Jersey.

Mead, M. 1930. Growing up in New Guinea. New York: William Morrow and Co.

Merton, R. K. 1940. Bureaucratic structure and personality. Social Forces, 18, 1-10.

Mills, C. A. 1942. Climatic effects on growth and development, with particular reference to the effects of tropical residence. American Anthropologist, 42, 1-14.

Mowrer, O. H. and C. Kluckhohn. 1943. Dynamic theory of personality. In Handbook of Personality and the Behavior Disorders, S. Mc V. Hunt, editor. The Ronald Press Co., New York

Murray, H. A. 1938. Explorations in Personality. New York: Oxford University Press.

Newman, H. H. 1940. Multiple human births. New York: Doubleday, Doran, and Co.

Rich, G. J. 1928. A biochemical approach to the study of personality. Journal of Abnormal and Social Psychology, 23, 158-175.

Sapir, E. 1934. The emergence of the concept of personality in a study of culture. Journal of Social Psychology, 5, 408-415.

Schilder, P. 1942. The sociological implications of neuroses. Journal of Social Psychology, 15, 3-23.

Sheldon, W. H. 1942. The varieties of temperament, a psychology of constitutional differences. New York: Harper and Brothers.

Sherif, M. 1935. A study of some social factors in perception. Archives of Psychology, no. 187.

Snyder, L. H. 1940. The principles of heredity. 2nd ed. New York. D. C. Heath and Co.

Woodworth, R. S. 1941. Heredity and environment. New York: Social Science Research Council, Bulletin 37.

Young, K. 1941. Personality and problems of adjustment. New York: F. S. Crofts and Co.

Zuckerman, S. 1933. Functional affinities of man, monkeys, and apes. New York: Harcourt Brace.

Cultural Shock: Theoretical and Applied

PAMELA J. BRINK / JUDITH M. SAUNDERS

The degree to which a patient is assessed as being in culture shock provides the nurse with a direction for nursing care. The foreign patient, flown into an American hospital for treatment, is more likely to suffer from severe culture shock than is the domestic patient. The first-admission patient may be severly affected by the transition from home to hospital. The long-term patient may be so socialized into the patient role that discharge-planning may be extremely threatening and the patient may require socialization into becoming a former patient.

Unlike the other articles in this section, which were directed primarily to the initial assessment of patients, this article speaks to the need for continuing assessment.

Culture shock is that malady that occurs in response to transition from one setting to another; in which the individual is placed in an unfamiliar situation where former patterns of behavior are totally ineffective; and in which basic cues for social intercourse are absent (Oberg 1954:1). The term *culture shock* covers all the feelings

An original paper. By permission of the authors.

and behaviors of people who have moved to unfamiliar countries. Although culture shock has been referred to in the literature quite frequently, the paper by Kalervo Oberg, delivered to the Women's Club in Rio de Janiero (Oberg 1954) has had the greatest impact on anthropology.

The purpose of this paper is to present culture shock within the context of the stress syndrome: stressors, response, and reconstitution. The primary task was to reformulate Oberg's original paper into a conceptual model that could be adapted by health professionals in contexts other than that of transition from country to country, since this phenomenon is infrequently encountered in hospitals or crises clinics in the United States. Life changes, whether positive or negative, have been found to be stress producing, either mildly or in the form of "shock" (Holmes and Holmes 1970, Holmes and Rahe 1967, Rahe 1972) involving either minor adjustments or death. If "normal" life changes can be conceived of as stressors necessitating both physiological and behavioral adaptations, what of the massive life change that occurs when an individual leaves home and country to live in an entirely foreign environment? The response can be termed a "shock" reaction, of interest to mental health personnel in relation to both primary and secondary prevention.

The paper is divided into two sections. The first deals with traditional culture shock phenomena from the stress-syndrome perspective. The second section applies the model to hospitalization as a form of attenuated culture shock. The authors propose that the overlay of culture shock upon a hospitalized patient simply adds to the patient's problems. If the health professional is aware of this phenomenon, he or she can take appropriate action to intervene early.

CULTURE SHOCK: A STRESS SYNDROME

The basic stressor involved in culture shock is the abrupt transition in residence from a familiar to an unfamiliar environment. Although the response to the stressor is both biological and emotional, the physiological aspects will not be discussed.

Abrupt transition from a familiar to an alien environment involves many major and minor differences in life styles and events, from a different taste of water to an inability to speak the language. To ennumerate every possible life change that might occur is not only exhausting but self-defeating, since not all individuals will experience all of the changes and others will experience changes not covered on the list. Therefore, the authors decided to group stressors into major categories. These categories were derived from a review of the literature, as well as from the author's experience with culture shock, but should not be considered exhaustive.

We must emphasize that stressors can be both positive and negative life changes, and that the individual may consider a change as either a loss or a gain to himself. However, change of any kind demands a readjustment, and multiple changes, no matter how positive, may result in a stress response, depending on individual coping styles.

Categories of Stressors

1) *Communication.* The primary stressor appears to be a changed system of communication, both verbal and nonverbal. In an entirely alien language system the individual finds himself playing the role of a deaf-mute. Although he still hears and sees, little meaning is ascribed to the verbal and nonverbal messages. Even when the language is known, tonal differences, colloquialisms, and other factors serve to obscure meaning. Systems of communication provide the major vehicle for obtaining and giving cues for behavior. In addition, communication provides feedback that enables us to modify our behavior to fit the situation. Lack of familiarity with portions of the system of communication is a impediment to appropriate behavior (Hall and Whyte 1960, Hall 1963, Watson and Graves 1966). Communication is certainly a primary stressor if the change in the communication system is one which impairs access to the meaning of behavioral cues.

2) *Mechanical Differences.* When one moves from one culture group to another, certain habitual activities and conveniences of daily living change. Utilities such as gas, electricity, telephone and water supply may not be available, or if available, only intermittently. Shopping for food and clothing change. Familiar modes of travel may not be available or may have difficult access. House types, furnishing, instruments, utensils, ornaments, or art work may have different functions or may demand a manual dexterity not previously encountered. Learning to manipulate the mechanical environment requires time and effort, and sometimes causes frustration.

3) *Isolation.* In addition to the isolation experienced in relation to the communication barrier, there remains the sense of isolation inherent in any situation totally populated by strangers. When an individual enters the field alone, or even with such significant others as spouse or nuclear family, the friendlessness and nonrelatedness to the immediate population is apparent. The distance between self and significant others is magnified and/or distorted. Dependence upon mail "from home" is increased. Making friends, becoming important or relevant to someone in the new situation is a time-consuming, often lonely task.

4) *Customs.* Customary, expected and/or anticipated patterns of behavior differ between host country and home and must be learned.

Although this stressor is directly related to the system of communication, the entire concept of reciprocal role relationships enters in. In particular, sex-linked role relationships must be established in the new setting. New role sets and systems of etiquette are often implicit rules of behavior rather than explicit. Class and status, kinship networks, and indeed the entire social structure, need to be understood to determine where one fits within the framework (Spradley and Phillips 1972).

5) *Attitudes and Beliefs.* Attitudes and values about human life and human behavior tend to distinguish one cultural group from another (Kluckhohn and Strodbeck 1961). Since belief systems are not necessarily explicit statements, they are more difficult to isolate and therefore easier to infringe upon. More insidious still, the field worker is often unaware of his own attitudes and belief systems prior to entering the field and reacts according to his belief system rather than that of the host country. This factor is far more critical for the applied scientist, but may slow, hamper, or totally destroy a setting for the field researcher.

Each of these five categories of stressors is external to the individual. Each stressor implies a change from a familiar series of life activities, and each individual change necessitates some sort of adaptation or adjustment in response. When all five categories are combined (are present at the same time) the impact is magnified and this certainly constitutes conditions capable of producing culture shock.

The Phases of Culture Shock

Oberg's original paper isolated and described four phases of culture shock and named the first phase the "Honeymoon Phase" (1954:3). The other three phases were described but not named. The following discussion is an attempt to name and extend Oberg's discussion.

Phase One. "The Honeymoon Phase" is marked by excitement. The desire to learn about the people and their customs is great; sightseeing is anticipated with pleasure; and getting to work and accomplishing all the goals envisioned at home provide the basis for this phase. Travelers, visiting dignitaries, and other temporary functionaries may never experience any other phase but this one.

Phase Two. "The Disenchantment Phase" generally does not begin until the individual has established residence, i.e., when he begins to become aware of the setting as his area of residence. This sense of awareness often is associated with the realization that one is "stuck here" and cannot get out of the situation. What was "quaint" may become aggravating. Simple tasks of living are time consuming because they must be done in a different way. This beginning awareness often results in frustration—either frustration because the indigenous population is too stubborn to see things your way or frustration because you can't see things their way and are constantly making social errors. Embarrassment coupled with feelings of ineptness attack self-image or self-concept.

Particular, individual styles of behavior are developed over the years through the principles of inertia and economy. Usually the individual is unaware of the operation of these principles and their effect to him. They form part of ethnocentrism: "The way I do things is the right way (and perhaps for some the only way) to do things." The disenchantment phase directly threatens ethnocentrism because the host country believes exactly the same way about its customs and sees no reason to change its ways. Phase two includes a reexamination of one's self from the vantage point of another set of values. In this phase failure often outweights success.

To this, add loneliness. No one knows you well enough to reaffirm your sense of self-worth. The distance from home is magnified. Home itself assumes the aura of Mecca—distant, unattainable, beautiful. This form of nostalgia for the past and the familiar seems to have two effects. Mail and visitors from home assume immense importance as a contact with people who believe in you and think you are important. To protect yourself from these feelings of loneliness and lack of self-esteem, you attack the presumed cause of these feelings—the host country. Feelings of anxiety and inadequacy are often expressed through depression, withdrawal, or eruptions of anger at frustration; or by seeking out fellow countrymen to the exclusion of the indigenous population. This period in the culture shock syndrome is the most difficult to live through and this is the period where people "give up and go home."

Phase Three. "The Beginning Resolution Phase." Oberg described this phase (1954:10-11) as the individual seeking to learn new patterns of behavior appropriate to the setting, attempting to make friends in the indigenous population, and becoming as much of a participant-observer as possible in the ceremonies, festivals, and daily activities of the new setting.

This phase seems to be characterized by the reestablishment of a sense of humor. Social errors no longer are devastating to the ego. The host culture no longer is considered all bad and home all wonderful. This phase seems to be facilitated greatly by the arrival of fellow countrymen who are "worse off" and need help. You can show off what you have learned, you are important because you are sought for advice, you feel needed by the newcomer.

At this point also, the individual becomes aware that things seem easier; friendships are being developed; home is still distant, but less relevant. Letters from home somehow seem peripheral to current interests and concerns. Letters to home become more superficial; explanation of what is becoming familiar would take up too much time. Current friendships have the same frame of reference for conversation, a frame of reference that is unknown at home.

Without really becoming aware of the process one slowly adapts to the new situation. Each small discovery, each small victory in learning the new rules is satisfying, and helps to restore one's sore and damaged ego.

Phase Four. "The Effective Function Phase." This means being just as comfortable in the new setting as in the old. Having achieved this phase, the individual will probably experience reverse culture shock when he returns home. Or, the individual may decide only to go home for visits, but make the new culture his own.

Coping with Culture Shock

Culture shock is diagnosed on the basis of behavior in phase two. Many people have lived and will continue to live in unfamiliar cultures without ever experiencing the discomforts of this phase; however, others will experience the stress of culture shock.

The disenchantment phase may be equivalent to the crisis phase in crisis theory or to the shock and disbelief phase of loss theory. For persons experiencing major difficulties in this phase, past coping mechanisms are ineffective, previous strategies are worse than useless, the future is bleak and hopeless, and the present is impossible to face. Resolution may terminate with the individual:

1. being healthier than in the past by adding to his arsenal of coping mechanisms;
2. being more rigid and/or ritualized in his coping mechanisms; or
3. emerging at an equivalent level of health.

If his resolution leads to fewer and more rigid adjustment methods, his discomfort may be increased and successful adjustment will be hampered. Three factors seem to enter into the effective resolution of this phase:

1. age
2. previous experience with changes in life style
3. generalized coping styles

Children, as a rule, adjust more readily to changes in their life space because they are still in the process of learning and are more flexible in what they think they can learn. Much of childhood learning is through participant-observations rather than through formal teaching methods. As one ages, habit patterns become more ingrained and there is diminished flexibility. Patterns of behavior become habitual, sometimes ritualized, without the individual being aware of the process. The principle of economy prevails. Once a behavior pattern is learned and becomes habitual, the individual no longer is aware of what he is doing. He puts certain things in the "back of his mind" so that he can devote his attention to new interests and new learnings. The principle of inertia assists this process. Once a behavior pattern is learned, comfortable, and out-of-awarness, an individual is loathe to give up the familiar (and now easy) way in order to learn a new way.

An individual exposed to repeated changes in life style over many years learns that the more rigid or closed his responses are, the more difficult it is to adapt to new situations. A person previously exposed to multiple changes, who has successfully adapted to these changes, should have less difficulty in resolving culture shock. Conversely, people with minimal experience in dealing with life changes may have a more difficult time since previous, possibly rigid coping mechanisms are entrenched.

Finally, regardless of age or past experience, an individual who has developed a *generalized* response to change should have greater adaptability than one who has developed specific (rigid or ritualized) responsive behaviors. The more generalized or flexible the coping mechanisms the more capable the individual should be of coping with change. This flexibility of coping strategies allows for a greater assimilation of simultaneous stressors without disintegration of the personality.

A person with inflexible coping patterns is in danger of damaged self esteem because the inability to use previously successful mechanisms leads to confusion about one's life style and values. At this juncture he becomes aware of the limited number of alternatives that are available to him. This individual probably has less potential for success in the resolution phase. He may attempt to create an isolated "little bit of home" in the foreign culture. He is less likely to learn the language and customs of the host country. He may consider himself and his countrymen superior to the "natives," and the host country "not quite as good" as home. For some, alcohol provides a refuge from the discomforts of this phase. These people may discover that their final resolution of culture shock places them in a lower position in the emotional health continuum than when they first entered the situation.

How long does phase two last? The length of the disenchantment phase varies according to the age, experience, flexibility, degree of difference between home and host country, and the reasons that brought the individual to the new setting. According to English and Coleman (1966) the Peace Corps volunteer experienced depression during the fourth month. They termed this period, which lasted from three to six months, "Crisis of Engagement"; this is equivalent to phase two of culture shock. The volunteer had received intensive language and cultural training prior to placement; he knew his period of tenure was two years; and he knew he was supposed to "help the natives." This pressure to produce, typical of Americans, placed an added burden on the volunteer, caused him to "start right away," and forced him to come to grips with the culture quite rapidly. The resistance to his best efforts to effect immediate change soon placed him in phase two.

Spradley and Phillips (1972:526) found that cultural readjustment was more difficult when the alternatives available in the new environment were greater than they were in the home environment. The problem stemmed more from the task of having to unlearn previous behaviors than from having to learn new behaviors.

HOSPITALIZATION AS CULTURE SHOCK

If the previous discussion has any validity for application, then culture shock should occur when the following criteria are present: bodily removal from one setting to another; existence of the five major environmental stressors; abrupt transition from one setting to another; and the need for planning the future in relation to the new setting. Movement from one culture to another or movement from one subculture to another appears to meet these criteria. In moving from one subculture to another, the five environmental stressors may be partially familiar, but new behavioral rules for each of the stressors must be acquired for the individual to be an acknowledged member of the new group. Also, in a subcultural transition, the individual might be less aware of the cause of his stress syndrome and of his reactions.

Subcultural transitions include changing residence; such as, from the east to the west coast; changing from a free citizen to a convict in a state or federal prison; and becoming a hospitalized patient. These examples can be termed "attenuated" culture shock situations and as a result may be difficult to recognize or understand.

Sociologists and anthropologists have used hospitals as field research laboratories. Their studies were based upon the assumption that hospitals meet all the requirements of a small society and, therefore, could be studied either as a separate culture or as a subculture of the largers society. In either case, the individual who associated himself with a hospital had to become acquainted with the hospital and its particular social system. For the person who became a patient, the added variable of having to take up residence in the hospital placed him in the position of exposure to culture shock.

People become "patients" in a variety of ways. The threat of illness (admission for diagnostic work-up, exploratory surgery) or the actual illness or injury are basic criteria for becoming a patient. Although the individual may not feel ill, fear of the unknown (final diagnosis) decreases his ability to cope with hospitalization as a change situation. The individual may be faced with no choice regarding hospitalization in the case of emergency surgery, injury (burns, automobile accidents) stroke, or heart attack. This abrupt transition from a free, independent, productive adult to an immobilized patient in a new setting can be seen as a stressor that requires not only adjustments in life style, but also in self-perception. Let us look briefly at the five environmental stressors which make this experience amenable to culture shock.

Communication. Although English is spoken predominantly, the patient must learn a new "language." Hospitals have their own communication systems. "Did you *void* this morning? When did you have your last BM? You are scheduled for EEG and when you get back we will call GYN for a work-up, then we will prep you for X-ray." Nurses continue to withhold information when patients ask about the medication they are receiving, saying either, "It will make you feel better" or "The doctor ordered it for you." Thirty-seven people may pop in and out of a patient's room in the space of a few hours, each with different uniforms and different tasks to perform, none of which is known to the patient.

Mechanical Differences. Hospital technology has made significant advances and requires learning on the part of both patients and new personnel. The patient must learn where to push a button to make the bed go up and down, how to make the side rails work, where the television remote control buttons are, how to operate the speaker to the nurses' station, and how to work the emergency signal in the toilet. Learning to use a bedpan rather than going to the toilet is in itself an adjustment. A simple cup of coffee during the morning must be requested, ordered, and brought by dietary personnel. Walking for exercise is restricted to the confines of the room and hall unless permission is obtained to go elsewhere. Add to these the adjustments that must be made to casts, traction, IV's, catheters, cardiac monitors, etc.

Customs. For most people, even medical personnel, becoming a patient for the first time requires learning a new role—that of being a patient. This new role involves learning to behave according to the standards set down by the new role set, usually the physicians, nurses, and other hospitals personnel. What familiar cues of social intercourse are available to the patient? The patient is expected to stay in bed even if he feels fine, and wear a hospital gown or his own sleepwear immediately upon admission even if it is in the middle of the day. He must rearrange his daily living schedule to fit into the hospital schedule. For the uninitiated, the customs of a hospital are foreign. Hospitalization involves learning both the hospital's customs and patient role behaviors.

Isolation. This stressor is immediately apparent in the case of the individual placed in isolation rooms. Patients are separated from family, friends, and work associates during most of the hospital day. Visiting hours and regulations further impede contact with relatives and friends. Activities of daily living occur within a situation comprised almost totally of strangers. The patient in the next bed may or may not be friendly, may or may not fill in the day with details of previous failures of medical science, may or may not remain throughout a particular hospitalization. Hospitalization is a lonely experience.

Attitudes and Beliefs. A certain mystique exists which hospital personnel tend to enhance—namely, that everyone in the hospital, except the patient, knows what is going on. The doctors and nurses know the diagnosis, know the treatment plan, and know the projected outcomes. "The patient is the last to know" is not as unusual as many think. The doctor or nurse is always right regardless of how the patient feels about the situation. The attitude of "the doctor knows best" or "that's what the doctor ordered" leaves little decision making to the patient. The patient is a low-status subordinate (Brink 1972) in the hospital hierarchy. When a patient asks a direct question about his disease or treatment plan and receives a vague or indirect non-answer, personnel are acting on the belief that it is to the patient's advantage to be uninformed or on the assumption that he does not have the right to know about himself or his disease process. Medical personnel maintain that patients are seeking help because health professionals know more about health than does the patient. Problems arise when health professionals do not see the need to teach their clients, but rather maintain the status relationship by keeping the patient in ignorance.

Culture Shock as Diagnosis. The "demanding patient" or the "difficult patient" might be diagnosed as phase two culture shock, if a previous knowledge of the patient reveals the behavior to be unusual. In looking over the hospitalization history, did the patient have a "honeymoon phase"? Did the patient ask innumerable questions? Was he interested in what was going on? How long did this phase last, if it occurred at all? What happened between admission and the time the demands began?

Knowing that all five stressors, in combination, exist from the time of admission, to which stressor is the patient responding? Is the patient angry because he is brought tea instead of coffee? (Mechanical.) Does the patient constantly call the nurse into his room on the pretext of needing a bedpan, when, in reality, he is afraid of being alone? (Isolation.) Does the patient say no to his medications or treatments? (Communication.) Does the patient continually ask unanswerable questions about his diagnosis and treatment? (Attitudes and Beliefs.) Does the patient insist on doing things "his way" regardless of the time and effort this imposes on the staff? (Customs.) Often the most difficult patient is responding to all five stressors. Here the patient is angry, scolds the staff about anything and everything, and is usually uncooperative or at best a time-waster. Hospitals with limited visiting hours reinforce feelings of loneliness and abandonment; anxiety and fear about the unexpected and unfamiliar increases; frustration with service, delays, and lack of information increases. All these feelings can be a result of culture shock.

When a patient stays long enough to learn the language, becomes familiar with technology and customs, becomes friendly with some of the staff, and can laugh and joke about some of the stressors, he should be in phase three. People usually are discharged at this time, if not before. When a patient is in phase three of culture shock, he is much easier to take care of since he is learning the patient role. The patient who has made some adjustments to previous hospitalizations should be an easier patient to care for in his future hospitalizations.

The more rapidly a patient achieves phase three, the more comfortable hospitalization will be for both staff and patient. When hospital personnel see a primary task in alleviating culture shock, fewer people will be discharged prematurely in phase two. If culture shock were understood better, then hospital personnel could intevene in all five of the common stressors in hospitalization. All personnel could receive in-service education on communication, attitudes towards services to the patient, information giving, and technology.

The major negative result of a successful resolution of culture shock, or phase four, is the patient who becomes so comfortable that he refuses to go home. Some patients have been known to develop new symptoms as the time of discharge approaches. Some mental patients in state hospitals have been so thoroughly socialized into the patient culture that "they can't make it on the outside." Hospitals cannot handle many phase four patients, and so must learn how to maintain patients in phase three and discharge them prior to phase four.

CONCLUSION

This paper has been presented as a conceptualization about culture shock and hospitalization that is amenable to research in either area; it provides a guide for direct intervention into "the problem patient," and for possible changes in administrative policies within the institution; it offers an alternative to a unidirectional approach to the assessment of patient care. If hospitals can be viewed as cultures, then hospitalization may result in culture shock. In order to reduce the chance of culture shock, the five environmental stressors can be reduced in kind and intensity through appropriate patient-care policies. Whether or not policy is changed, the personal contact that occurs between hospital personnel and patient can be directed toward alleviating the response to the stressors through knowledge that the stressors exist and of how they may be reduced.

REFERENCES

Brink, Pamela J., "Natural Triad in Health Care," *American Journal of Nursing* 72 (1972):897-99.

English, Joseph T. and Joseph G. Coleman, "Psychological Adjustment Patterns of Peace Corps Volunteers," *Psychiatric Opinion* 3 (1966):29-35.

Hall, Edward T., "A System of Notation of Proxemic Behavior," *American Anthropologist* 65 (1963):1003-26.

Hall, Edward T. and William Foote Whyte, "Intercultural Communication, A Guide to Men of Action," *Human Organization* 19 (1960):5-12.

Holmes, T. Stephenson and Thomas H. Holmes, "Short Term Intrusion into the Life Style Routine," *Journal of Psychosomatic Medicine* 14 (1970):121-32.

Holmes, Thomas H. and Richard H. Rahe, "The Social Readjustment Rating Scale," *Journal of Psychosomatic Medicine* 11 (1967):213-18.

Kluckhohn, Florence R. and Fred L. Strodbeck, *Variations in Value Orientations.* Elmsford, New York: Row Peterson and Company, 1961.

Oberg, Kalervo, *Culture Shock.* Indianapolis: Bobbs-Merrill Co., Inc., 1954.

Rahe, R. H., "Subject's Recent Life Changes and their Near-Future Illness Reports," *Annals of Clinical Research* 4 (1972):250-65.

Spradley, James P., and Mark Phillips, "Culture and Stress: A Quantitative Analysis," *American Anthropologist* 74 (1972):518-29.

Watson, O. Michael and Theodore E. Graves, "Quantitative Research in Proxemic Behavior," *American Anthropologist* 68 (1966):971-85.

Methods and Strategies

Nurses act, react, and interact with people every day of their lives. Each piece of interaction, whether with patients, family, or friends, occurs in a cultural context and can be viewed as cultural data. For this reason, the method of participant observation becomes the method of choice in data collection about patients. Looking, listening, asking questions, and taking notes are the basic tools for acquiring information about another person's culture. In fact, this method of data collection is exactly the one that nurses use in interaction with patients in relation to their current illness situation; the researcher, on the other hand, is collecting data for its possible future relevance to the problem. For the one, the purpose is immediate problem solving; for the other the purpose is to generalize. The techniques remain essentially the same.

Participant observation is based on the premise that the research subject, whether an individual or a group, is a whole made up of a variety of interacting parts. Each part has a definite function in relation to the other parts of the system, so that if there is a dysfunction in one part it will affect the other parts of the system most closely allied to it. For the participant observer, nothing is irrelevant. Every piece of information fits in somewhere eventually. Careful and complete notetaking is a necessity for this type of research since the researcher cannot remember all of the myriad or minute details that he experiences. Recording on the spot or immediately after an interaction prevents memory loss. The data that are collected are rich in meaning and feeling.

Participant-observation requires that the researcher participate (as far as possible) in the life of his subjects. The researcher must find some appropriate role which is acceptable to the people with whom he is interacting. In the United States, there is a distinct role of researcher, one that is understood and reacted to—sometimes negatively. The participant-observer, more than any other social scientist, pries into the affairs of others and must guard against invasion of privacy and the possible embarrassment of his subjects. For this reason, published findings should not include identifying information.

Because of the negative reaction of people to being studied, the participant-observer usually selects a role for himself other than researcher. The nurse-researcher has a ready-made role for herself—the role of nurse—which is the envy of other social scientists. The nurse interested in participant-observation simply has to present herself as a possible employee to gain entry, establish herself in an acceptable social role, and participate in the life and work of that particular health agency. The article by Gale, in the list of recommended readings, exemplifies this form of role taking. Gale was interested in nursing from the point of view of the nurses' aide. She, therefore applied to a hospital to become a nurses' aide, was accepted, and pursued participant-observation from that vantage. Or the scientist can take the role of patient, as in the Rosenhan article. Regardless of the role taken, the researcher must become the person he says he is.

Participant-observation requires direct contact with the research subjects and cannot be accomplished long distance. When the researcher wants to understand the subject, from the subject's point of view, participant observation is the method of choice. Interviews and questionnaires, the basic tools of the social scientist, elicit what people say they think and do, but cannot elicit what a person actually does in a situation. The method of participant-observation confirms or denies what a person says he would do in a given situation.

Participant-observation is the study of human behavior by looking, listening, asking questions, and attempting to live the life of the subject according to the rules of the group, with as little disruption as possible. Every behavior, every human act, has an explanation or a reason. The participant-observer not only observes the action but searches for the rationale behind the action, and attempts to place the action within its appropriate context.

As a research method, participant-observation is a data-collection technique. The tool used is the researcher himself. The more sensitive the researcher is to behavioral cues and the more objective he is in his observations, the greater the possibility that he will not distort his reporting of what he sees. The success of the technique is totally dependent upon the researcher. As a participant in the cultural context, however, the researcher is apt to make enemies as well as friends, be rejected as well as accepted, and become subjective as well as objective. Just as the nurse uses herself as a therapeutic tool in nurse-patient interactions, the researcher uses himself as a sensitive instrument in participant-observation.

Participant-observation is a research method that fits easily within the process of nursing assessment. Byerly's article describes the uses of participant-observation in a hospital setting, and some of the difficulties of the nurse-researcher in a familiar setting. The list of references she provides should be read by all nurses interested in this method of research, and are considered an addendum to the list of recommended readings.

The articles by Byerly and Ragucci exemplify Osborne's contention that nursing can add to anthropological science. Both have taken the basic research method of anthropology and applied it to a nursing problem. As a result, both have contributed to medical anthropology as well as to transcultural nursing. Ragucci uses participant-observation in urban anthropology. She examined health and illness beliefs and customs of Italian-American women in a self-contained community within a large American city, and found differences and similarities in the health practices over three generations.

Another example of participant-observation as a basic research technique is Rosenhan's fascinating article, "On Being Sane in Insane Places." When the article first appeared in *Science*, it raised a furor in the psychiatric community—many disagreed with Rosenhan's findings. However, psychiatry is an imprecise field, as was clearly shown. One important finding in this article is that many people, health professionals included, relate to other people according to their role. When people are admitted to a hospital and are labeled "patient," the staff interact with them as patients and do not question the validity of the label. This is true not only in psychiatric settings but in general medical institutions as well. Once the patient has been labeled, staff frequently respond to the label rather than to the person.

A valid field of inquiry in transcultural nursing incorporates the research and theory of physical anthropology. The brief report by Kasselman is an example of the interdigitation between nursing and physical anthropology; the surprising finding that there was little difference in delivery patterns and reproductive efficiency between Negro and Caucasian women when the class factor is controlled for is further substantiated in the paper on hysterectomy by Williams.

She, too, found fewer differences (between Mexican-American and Anglo women) than she had anticipated when she controlled for class and generation. Further work into nutritional variables remains to be done, but such an initial exploration is vital to our understanding of intercultural variation.

"Unleashing the Untrained" is the last article in this section. Teaching is a part of nursing and some of the unexpected findings described by Meyers could be duplicated over and over again in many nursing contexts. The wry humor of this article is needed in nursing.

The one area that is missing in this section, vitally needed in transcultural nursing, is the research method of ethnolinguistics or ethnographic semantics. The discovery of an individual's culture by examining his language is critical to the field. For this reason the book by Spradley and McCurdy has been added to the list of recommended readings in the hope that this method of data collection might be incorporated into nursing research. The discovery of how people categorize their illnesses provides insight into health beliefs and practices. The article by Louie in the next section is a description of findings that may have been collected through this method. As the field of transcultural nursing develops, the research methods will become more available in the literature.

RECOMMENDED READINGS

Gale, Charlotte, "Walking in the Aide's Shoes," *American Journal of Nursing* 73, No. 4 (1973):628-631.

Glaser, Barney G., and Anselm L. Strauss, *The Discovery of Grounded Theory: Strategies for Qualitative Analysis.* Chicago: Aldine-Atherton, 1967.

Pelto, Perti J., *Anthropological Research: The Structure of Inquiry.* New York: Harper & Row, Publishers, 1970.

Schatzman, Leonard, and Anselm L. Strauss, *Field Research: Strategies for a Natural Sociology.* Englewood Cliffs, N.J.: Prentice-Hall, Inc., 1973.

Schwartz, Morris, and Charlotte Schwartz, "Problems in Participant Observation," *American Journal of Sociology* 60 (1955):343-353.

Spradley, James P., and David W. McCurdy, *The Cultural Experience: Ethnography in Complex Society.* Prospect Heights, IL: Waveland Press, Inc., 1972 (reisssued 1988).

Whiting, John W. M., Irvin L. Child, and William W. Lambert, *Field Guide for the Study of Socialization.* New York: John Wiley & Sons, 1966.

The Nurse-Researcher as Participant-Observer in a Nursing Setting

ELIZABETH LEE BYERLY

As a research strategy, participant-observation was developed by anthropologists for use in small isolated communities. The method is equally applicable to hospitals as the article by Byerly shows.

Nurses, by the very nature of their nursing, are participant-observers. Nurses participate in nurse-patient interactions, within the health team, within health agencies, and in the community. At the same time, nurses are observers of what is happening around them. Byerly describes how the nurse as a participant-observer can objectify what she sees and hears, can put that information into context, and can analyze the meaning of the information. As a technique, participant observation has immediate applicability for nursing. Although this article is highly sophisticated, the list of references provided by Byerly, as well as the recommended readings at the end of this section, can be used for further discussion of this technique.

 Thanks are due to the author for substantial revision of the previously published paper "The Nurse-Researcher as Participant-Observer in a Nursing Setting," published in *Nursing Research* 18, No. 3 (1969):230-36.

Any research involving face-to-face relationships between a human scientist and a human subject necessitates both participation and observation; therefore, most human behavioral research involves participant-observation whether or not the scientist is aware of and in conscious control of the method (Pearsall 1965). As a general method in human behavioral science research, participant-observation has enjoyed increasing popularity in recent years. Pearsall (1965:37) noted three distinct and analytically separate aspects of participant-observation: 1) as a role, implying reciprocal roles, 2) as a body of techniques for gathering detailed information, ranging "from the eclecticism of the anthropologist to the parsimonious elegance of the experimental psychologist," and 3) as a methodology for obtaining maximal knowledge and understanding of human behaviors in the sociocultural and psychosocial context.

This paper addresses participant-observation as a role, specifically that of a nurse-researcher employing the method in a health care setting where nursing role behavior is the focus. In so doing, techniques and methodological considerations will be seen to influence and be influenced by the participant-observer's relationship with the persons studied.

McCall and Simmons (1969), in the preface to their reader on issues in participant-observation, list five characteristics of the method which they state as reasons for a lack of systematization and codification, resulting in the method being least often and least adequately taught. These characteristics may also be viewed as influential in choice and performance of the role as participant-observer. Briefly, following McCall and Simmons, it may be said that

1. participant-observation is not a single method but rather a characteristic style of research which makes use of a number of methods and techniques—observation, informant interviewing, document analysis, respondent interviewing, and participation with self-analysis;
2. participant-observation is intentionally unstructured in research design; in refusing preconceived hypotheses, participant-observers do not "employ *a priori* standardizations of concepts, measures, samples, and data, but rather seek to discover and revise these" as they learn more about the people or organizations studied;
3. the resulting data are typically qualitative rather than quantitative;
4. participant-observation is a relatively expensive procedure in the time required for active field involvement by the researcher; and

5. practical problems met by the researcher in his relationships with the subjects of the study require considerable thought and human relations work.

Similar descriptions, advantages, and disadvantages of participant observation have been discussed in the increasing publications on this method. (Pelto, 1970; Whiting and Whiting, 1973; Dean, Eishhorn & Dean, 1969)

PARTICIPANT-OBSERVATION AS ROLE

The nurse-researcher who chooses participant observation as the general method for obtaining behavioral data from and about human subjects in their natural setting also selects, as a matter of course, an interpretation of the role which will best serve her research ends. Pearsall (1965:38) suggests a continuum for the master role of participant-observer: (1) complete observer, (2) observer-as-participant, (3) participant-as-observer, and (4) complete participant.

Limitations of complete observation are inherent in the necessity for complete physical (undetected observation) or verbal withdrawal from the study setting. Not only do such withdrawals raise ethical questions, they eliminate the opportunity for two-way verbal communication which might clarify or confirm what has been observed. Objectivity is obtained, but completeness is not. At the other extreme, the complete participant risks problems in both moral and scientific defense of his choice of method. He may gain more complete experience of the subject's sociocultural milieu, but he loses much objectivity in the process. Caudill (1958) has reported his problems in using concealed identity during field research in a mental hospital.

For the observer-as-participant, observation takes precedence either by choice or from a necessity to engage in numerous brief contacts with many persons (Pearsall 1965:38). While this role is limited in opportunities for obtaining knowledge of the total situation, it has the advantage of presenting a more detached image and may result in use of the observer as a "sounding board" for feelings and opinions that might not be expressed to someone more intimately involved in the immediate physical situation.

The participant-as-observer is able, by virtue of closer interpersonal relationships with his informants, to obtain a wider range of information from multiple sources. Such participation places the observer "in the midst of social and cultural activity, though he must inevitably remain to some degree a perpetual and unassimilable stranger" (Pearsall 1965:38). Participation tends to increase and become more sociable. In so doing, "it takes time and energy, often at the expense of objective observation and systematic recording" (Pearsall 1965:38). Significant items may be overlooked as the observer becomes more of an integral part in the observed activity.

Both observer and observed tend to vacillate between the observer-as-participant and participant-as-observer roles. Pearsall (1965:38) notes that people tend to handle the vaguely disturbing presence of the researcher by pulling him into their ranks, where he is subject to their sanctions, and then pushing him out again when his behavior becomes too threatening. The participant-observer himself also vacillates in his attempt to protect himself against loss of rich and pertinent data and against personal over-involvement. He handles his dilemma by increasing or decreasing the amount of participation according to his evaluation of the demands of the moment.

Influence of the Fieldworker on the Data

Fieldwork has given strong support to participant-observation as a means not only for collecting raw data but for checking and rechecking these data over time. Schwartz and Schwartz (1955) describe the process of participant-observation as one of registering, interpreting, and recording; it is unavoidably retrospective when the researcher looks at data in the context of the total field. In retrospect, the observer tries to recreate the social field in his imagination, in all its dimensions, on a perceptual and feeling level.

When fieldwork is used as a research method, Quint (1967) notes, the data are collected and analyzed by human observers, thus the participant-observer becomes the instrument. She emphasizes the necessity "to recognize and use one's inner conflicts and biases as an essential part of the data being collected and analyzed." Schwartz and Schwartz (1955:352) assume that bias is a universal phenomenon. "The observer can and does know what his biases are, and knowing what they are, he can by specifying them, prevent distortion of his observations." The individual's frame of reference influences the selections he makes from the phenomena and determines how and what is observed. Because effective involvement is a function of the observer's experience, awareness, and personality, and the way these are integrated with the particular social situation, he has to contend with his feelings as part of the data (Schwartz and Schwartz 1955:350). Vidich (1955) says the participant-observer must be skeptical of himself in all data-gathering situations. Not only does the fieldworker need to become aware of his own strength and weaknesses in observational style, but he should practice observing and recording events in order to discover his observational biases and to develop more systematic techniques of recall (Pelto 1970:92).

The participant-observer, of necessity, assumes reciprocal roles with his subjects in the field situation. Florence Kluckhohn (1940) notes the need for assuming a general role or roles, which have definition in terms of the community's set of organized statuses, that influence the quantity and quality of the data to an unknown degree. The researcher must determine how group members define him, and "in particular, whether or not they believe certain kinds of information and events should be kept hidden from him" (Becker 1958). Recognition that such influence does occur is acknowledged by the observer as he reports his findings.

Anthropologists, who have immersed themselves in the culture of the human groups they study, are familiar with problems of maintaining the necessary objectivity in data collection and analysis while living and working in close association with their subjects over a considerable period of time. Read's (1965) sensitive portrayal of his experience in New Guinea is an unusually frank discussion of such a role. Laura Bohannan's novel, *Return to Laughter* (Bowen 1964), is remarkable in its introspection of a field worker's life among a tribal people and its depiction of pitfalls and uncertainties in the relationships with them.

Most field researchers acknowledge their possible influence on the data obtained. Some do so in sufficient detail to permit others to recognize the existence of possible limitations (Spiro 1958). Such limitations are important to consider for at least two reasons: (1) to help other investigators realize that it is not possible to achieve total success in obtaining purely objective data in a field study, and (2) to emphasize a need for some recognition of similar limiting factors when evaluating data and conclusions from all type of human behavioral studies.

The investigator's sex may affect success in obtaining certain types of information. If restrictions are imposed by the group on the anthropologist's contact with either men or women, the data may be affected. Male anthropologists may describe men's initiation rites in detail but may find it difficult or impossible to obtain accurate information about women's initiation ceremonies; the reverse may be true for female researchers. A linguist, unaware that men and women speak different dialects within a certain living group, acquires only a partial knowledge of the language of that group when he uses only male informants. As Reisman notes (Bowen 1964:XVI) women sometimes have an advantage in fieldwork because they have access to the private worlds of women as a member of their sex, but are also, by virtue of their occupational role and the assertiveness allowed, able to penetrate such male worlds as magic and statecraft.

Limitations and advantages of a related sort obtain for a behavioral scientist studying complex societies. A nurse-researcher studying the behavior of nurses in a health-care setting may avoid the "culture shock" experienced by a non-nurse under similar circumstances; he or she may be sensititve to certain aspects of nursing behavior which a non-nurse may not notice or not fully comprehend. On the other hand, a nurse may overlook pertinent details which are part of the cognitive orientation of a nurse, details that might be immediately obvious to a non-nurse.

In seeking to maintain objectivity, the nurse participant-observer may find it necessary to withdraw, physically and/or mentally, from involvement in the immediate behavioral situation. This often is accomplished quite simply by moving back a few feet from the main scene of action. In other instances, the observer may find it necessary to leave the setting completely.

This writer first experienced vacillation between observer-as-participant and participant-as-observer roles during a social anthropological study of hospital nurses as they sought to create conditions which allowed them to function with relative freedom in their roles. The study, using a general systems approach, focused on methods of handling potentially disruptive situations and identified behavioral and ecological factors which contributed to increase in tension and threatened a "steady state" equilibrium in the work milieu. It also examined behavioral mechanisms employed to reduce tension and threat to that equilibrium. The effect of interpolation of the nurse-researcher into the hospital ward situation was tension-producing to varying degrees for the nurses (Byerly 1970).

DILEMMAS IN DEFINING THE NURSE PARTICIPANT-OBSERVER ROLE

Although it is obvious that the skills and techniques of the individual play a considerable part in how the actual research role develops, there are certain dilemmas presented by the role which must be considered by any member of a profession engaging in field research focusing on members of that profession. For persons already experienced in field research, the problems will appear familiar; for those about to embark on such a study, recognition of their existence helps in defining the researcher's role in response to informants' expectations.

The nurse participant-observer encounters three main dilemmas in the selected role: (1) objectivity versus subjectivity, (2) preservation of the scientific integrity of the study and/or protection of the rights of individuals who are the subjects of research, and (3) nonintervention into the activities of the study group versus intervention which risks changing the course of the findings.

Objectivity/Subjectivity

The question of objectivity in behavioral research arises when the researcher places herself/himself in any face-to-face encounter with the subjects in the study. When data are collected solely by means of a questionnaire or an interview which is structured and restricted as to content, the investigator has limited contact with the subjects and objectivity is more easily obtained. It is possible in this situation to define oneself as "researcher" and to play this part as the informants expect it to be played. The active participant-observer, on the other hand, is placed in numerous interaction situations over a considerable period of time. As the study population come to know the researcher better, he/she finds himself/herself playing many roles other than researcher. Some of these multiple roles assist in obtaining data which cannot be secured in the research role alone; others hinder the data-gathering. The researcher will likely find herself/himself shifting between the roles of participant-as-observer and observer-as-participant (Pearsall 1965). Conscientiously recorded field notes provide the researcher with an opportunity to reflect on the roles played, on how the investigator's own behavior might have affected the response obtained, and on how, in turn, this response affected her/his feelings and subsequent attempts to elicit information.

The nurse participant-observer may find herself/himself in several differently perceived roles even as researcher; these depend on the differing expectations of the persons studied. The nurse-researcher can be seen as an expert of sorts in nursing, or as someone to be asked for advice on how to solve problems. The investigator may serve as a sounding-board, and, sometimes, as an object of catharsis. The question of unknown motives of informants, collective and individual, often arises; unwillingness to be placed in a false position tends to put the researcher on guard. This forces evaluation of the objectivity or subjectivity of the researcher's own behavior in encounters with the study group. In most instances, the role of neutral observer will be sufficient; occasionally simple answers to questions are enough. Each incident should be handled in its total context.

Scientific Integrity/Protection of Rights of Individuals

Protection of rights of individuals is a major concern in behavioral science research (Abdellah 1967; American Nurses' Association Committee on Research Studies 1968; American Anthropological Association 1973). Abdellah (1967:318) emphasizes the responsibility of the investigator for obtaining consent and maintaining confidentiality in behavioral research. The researcher has both a legal and moral responsibility to inform the subjects, in terms they can understand, of the purpose of the study and how the information will be used. In longitudinal field studies, the original hypotheses may be revised and refocused as new data arise in the course of the investigation. Because of the flexibility inherent in such studies, the researcher is faced with the question of the extent of the original implied consent. Here the investigator must be guided by professional judgment to protect the rights of individual subjects, while still maintaining integrity of the research.

Anonymity and protection of the privacy of informants can be managed satisfactorily if caution is used in reporting of findings. The investigator must decide if and how to handle information given in confidence which is, nonetheless, highly pertinent, but which cannot be used without violating that confidence. In addition, some data are so specific that they point to an easily identifiable individual. Information regarding a certain employee not only places him at risk but may also reflect on others in the same setting. The observer must weigh possible actions of persons in power and authority positions in the organization or social group and decide whether the knowledge held is crucial to the final reporting of the research.

Behavior should be reported without judgment on the part of the investigator. It is, however, human nature to judge according to one's own values; some readers tend to criticize the behavior of others in light of their own expectations rather than on the basis of scientific research. There is no question that behavioral research may be a threat to the subjects; therefore, decisions must be made as to the relative importance of the subjects' rights to privacy as they relate to goals of the study.

Intervention/Nonintervention

The nurse researcher has at some time experienced socialization into the nursing subculture as a practitioner of nursing. A third major dilemma is whether to intervene when information has been obtained which appears directly pertinent to the welfare of a patient. Occasions arise when the researcher may feel forced to make a nursing judgment, even though the primary goal of the study does not involve patient care. Placed in a position where she/he must make some response, the nurse participant-observer finds that a blank stare and noncommittal answer are seldom sufficient.

Anthropologists tend to identify with those whom they may call "my people." If they become concerned with problems of the persons studied they may wish to "improve the situation." The ensuing role conflict results not just from an inability to do anything about the situation, but rather from the knowledge that if it were not for self-imposed restrictions for research purposes, intervention with the appropriate authority might bring about a change. Conflicting obligations to hospital unit nurses and to hospital nursing administrators are similar to the dilemmas described by Olesen and Whittaker (1968) in their relationships with students and faculty.

Personal values of the nurse-researcher actually may pose problems as she/he observes and evaluates the fairness or unfairness of the treatment of patients or employees and feels powerless to act. It is not uncommon to receive subtle suggestions from "my people" to do something to change the situation. If no pressure is placed on the investigator by the administration during the course of study, there may be a few expressions of hope that something of benefit will come to the organization.

The participant-observer becomes aware that the human subjects chosen for study are playing a considerable part in determining the flexible parameters of the research role. The ultimate role chosen and the manner in which decisions are made to deal with dilemmas of that role depend on what sort of reciprocal behavior has developed between the observer and the study group.

ATTEMPTS BY ONE STUDY GROUP TO DEFINE THE ROLE OF THE RESEARCHER

Goffman (1959, 1961) has discussed methods by which individuals in social interaction attempt to control the impressions others may receive of the situation. Participant-observation during anthropological field research in a community general hospital provided an opportunity to observe the behavior of selected nurses as they attempted to define for themselves the role of a nurse-researcher. They probed for clues and they sought to determine their own roles in response to that of the investigator. One of the first questions asked by a licensed practical nurse was, "Are we going to be guinea pigs?" Another nurse observed, "She is an anthropologist and we are her primitive culture." At the conclusion of a nursing staff dinner, one registered nurse asked the investigator, "Well, was our behavior all right?" Numerous comments were made in speculation of the final disposition of the data: "Miss B is writing a huge book, and we are all going to be in it!"

Presentation of the Researcher Role to the Study Group

The investigator first met with nursing staff on the study unit in two brief sessions on consecutive days, in order to contact as many as possible at the same time. She presented herself as an anthropologist who also happened to be a nurse; she was already known to several persons in the hospital as a nurse and nothing seemed to be gained by attempting to conceal this fact from personnel on the unit.

During the initial contact, staff were told that the researcher would be making observations over a period of several months, would be interested in the kinds of job activities they performed, and would ask them questions periodically. The investigator told them she would be present quite a bit of the time, and, although she knew it would be impossible for them to ignore her presence, she preferred they try to consider her "part of the furniture" and go about their duties as usual. The following illustrates some of the mechanisms employed by nurses in their attempts to define the unfamiliar role of a field researcher, and describes the tactics they used to place the investigator in a more predictable role.

Reactions to the Data-Gathering Activities

The first active data-gathering occurred in the form of time-and-activity studies on the nursing unit. There was a general air of adventure among the personnel and they volunteered a considerable amount of information about their activities, although they did exhibit occasional uneasiness at having their exact actions and whereabouts recorded at frequent, regular intervals. The researcher had explained the purpose of this part of the study: the gathering of background data to gain some idea of the daily routine, who did what, and where on the nursing unit it was done. The group was not entirely unfamiliar with activity studies, having participated in one conducted by nursing administration during the previous year.

Even at this early stage, the researcher noted an attempt to keep her at a certain distance; this was manifested in subtle warnings expressed in joking or teasing behavior. "Ah, here comes the spy." "Are you here again making everyone uneasy?" "Miss B is looking to see if we really cut the mustard. She assures us it won't make any difference in our jobs." As the study progressed other attempts to control became evident.

Efforts were made almost immediately to draw the observer into, and place her within, the group. On the second day of contact she was invited to a staff dinner held the same evening, "So you can get to know us better." She was invited by the nurses to join them on coffee and lunch breaks. First-naming, a common practice among the registered nurses on the unit, was extended in both reference and address of the observer. On the other hand, the licensed practical nurses, nurse aids, and orderlies, who frequently used either the last name or diminution of the last name as terms of reference and address among themselves, employed the same formal terms with the researcher as they reserved for most of the registered nurses or administrative personnel in the hospital.

Considerable deference was shown the observer by the nursing staff. Upon entering a conference room, she was always offered a chair, even if someone had to leave the room to obtain one. Conversely, when she offered a stool at the nursing station to someone who was standing, it was invariably refused. At a staff picnic, when she offered to refill their coffee cups, two licensed practical nurses protested to the observer, "We should be waiting on you." Although this solicitous behavior diminished after a period of weeks, it continued to some degree throughout the study.

Most registered nurses appeared to conclude that the writer was looking for problems, although this was not the case, nor had it been so stated to them. A sampling of comments revealed: "We were looking for you this morning. We had all kinds of problems." "We really had a crisis yesterday." "We were all in a bad mood this morning." "Miss B is writing a full length novel. I hope you say something about the fact that the elevator is never available when we need it." "Come to coffee with me. I need your moral support." Some nurses came to the investigator to describe specific problems: "Now this is a good example of why such-and-such (policy or procedure) doesn't work." In such instances, the researcher tried to present a sympathetic ear, but refrained from making any judgmental response.

Suggestions that the observer's time could be put to better use also offered options to do something about problems which concerned the nursing staff: "Where were you this morning when we were going crazy with all these patients? We could have used an extra nurse." "We could have used you yesterday as a ward secretary. She didn't come to work." "I'm glad you had a chance to help to be a ward secretary today. Now you can see how busy we can be at the desk when she isn't here."

Reaction to the participant-observer's occasional offers of assistance with patient care were varied. Although some personnel allowed her to help, others seemed to communicate, usually nonverbally, that her assistance was neither needed nor desired. To help with such an activity as bedmaking had seemed to the nurse participant-observer to be an easy and natural way to observe basic activities and enter into informal conversations. She was surprised at the amount of resistance to these offers and decided not to assist actively with patient care because of this response.

On the other hand, she was asked by the charge nurse to perform some clerical work at the nursing station: "Could I impose on you to answer the telephone for a few moments while I make rounds with the doctor?" "Would you do me a favor, Liz, and copy this assignment sheet?" "How would you like to be ward secretary today?" Such incidents happened only rarely, but when the observer agreed to help, the entire staff seemed to accept as appropriate this less-threatening form of participation in ward activities.

Some questioning by the observer drew answers from the nurses which seemed to reflect a concern that she might be criticizing their nursing practice: "I suppose we should, but we just don't have time." "I was taught to do it another way, but this is the way they want to do it here."

The observer found that she served as audience for a number of complaints which reflected dissatisfaction with circumstances in which the nurses had to execute their roles. For some of these she was a sounding board. Some less-direct performances seemed staged for her benefit, perhaps because the individuals found it too uncomfortable to state their feelings more directly. Nurses who appeared to fear they might have been indiscreet in expressing feelings and opinions to her reacted in one or both of two ways: avoidance of her for some time afterward or, later, asking her to say nothing of what she had been told.

On occasion there were less subtle sanctions and attempts to control the research activities. Interviews during the early part of the research were granted and participated in with some enthusiasm. Later in the study, appointments for some interviews were put off because the nurses were "too busy to spend time until the census goes down." Scheduled appointments, though granted without protest, began late or were sometimes interrupted in the middle because the nurse had some duty to perform. The reason given for any reduction in cooperation with the study most frequently was the plea that the individual was too busy with her nursing activities. In such instances the researcher did not push the effort. It appears that there is a time limit beyond which tolerance of research activities may be markedly diminished and the wise investigator is alert to cues which suggest the efforts should be postponed or terminated altogether. Most field workers recognize the point beyond which further time in the field may add little to what data have already been obtained.

Few overt expressions of hostility were directed toward the observer; these were for the most part impersonal in nature and associated with the individual's displeasure with the current scene. In any field situation, it is important that the researcher avoid acting defensive or suspicious of responses to her/his presence or to the purpose of the research. The behaviors illustrated here were sufficiently patterned to permit the conclusion that they lay within the normal range of expected responses in similar instances. In later analysis of the data the writer found that field notes containing such examples were of help in developing hunches which aided in interpretation of certain observed behaviors.

Recording of the Field Notes

Observations were made at random times throughout the progress of the study. This activity covered longer periods of time at the beginning than later in the research when data collection was more focused. Field notes provided a record of observations throughout the study. They served as accounts of temporal and spatial relationships of the actors; actors' stated values and related actions; the hospital sociocultural setting within which the actors performed; and general nursing role behavior in a variety of situations.

Some notes were recorded during the time an activity was occurring; others were written as soon as possible after the investigator left the scene of action. Additional comments were placed on magnetic tape; these were recorded while the day's events were still fresh in the observer's mind. Taped comments, though valuable records of the investigator's personal reactions to observed situations, as manifested by vocal tones and inflections during the recording, were unwieldy and time-consuming to transcribe and were discontinued during early stages of the research.

Decisions about when and where to make notations were related to the formality or informality of the immediate situation. The investigator found that she and the subjects were most comfortable when noticeable writings was restricted to formal situations such as interviews, patient reports, administrative meetings, or routine observations of nursing activities. In less formal settings such as meals, coffee breaks, incidental conversations, or social gatherings, recording was delayed and occurred out-of-sight of the actors. When the nurses appeared uneasy or the researcher thought her writing might be threatening, taking of notes was reserved until later. When notations were made on the scene, they were executed either openly within full view of the actors, or less openly by holding the notebook in the lap below the edge of a desk or table. At no time was the activity intended to appear surreptitious. The investigator did not discuss the contents of the notes with the informants; only one nurse asked when she might see the results of the time-and-activity studies, and she appeared satisfied with the explanation that they would not be analyzed until later.

Fortunately, the anthropologist became more adept at recalling conversations and actions as the study progressed. Improvement of this ability was coincident with collection of the more sensitive data, and proved an advantage in intimate conversations with some of the nurses at a time when note-taking would have been inhibiting.

Field notes served as the reservoir of data from which hypotheses were inductively derived. Notes were oriented intially toward a general examination of the hospital system; subsequently, they centered on nursing role with the purpose of identifying aspects of role behavior which appeared to contribute to system stability. As the study progressed, it became possible to focus on methods of control used by the nurses as they sought to reduce discrepancies between values and goals and the reality of the situation within which they performed. Their handling of the researcher and her participant-observer role was a part of this control.

THE PARTICIPANT-OBSERVER ROLE IN NURSING RESEARCH AND CLINICAL PRACTICE

As a nursing research method, participant observation may range from a complete ethnography of one health care sociocultural system; to using the technique as a complement to projective techniques in analyzing effectiveness of health care in an agency; to an observation of interactive behavior in a specifically structured patient-care situation. Selection between macro or micro approaches to participant observation of human behavior depends on the scope and purpose of the investigation; it is far from an "either-or" matter, and the researcher may elect to use both approaches at different points during a study.

Participant-observation as used by Van de Bittner (1973) proved to be a valuable adjunct to semantic differential and open-ended questionnaire techniques during an in-depth analysis of health care delivery in two walk-in clinics. While the semantic differential provides more objectivity, it is also more dependent on language, one source of error due to variability of interpretation (Webb 1966). Participant-observation can be used to provide behavioral data which are then compared with written and verbal responses.

Growing numbers of nurse-anthropopololgists are doing research in all areas of human behavioral and clinical nursing interests: maternal-child, psychosocial, physiological, community health, pharmacological, and health care administration, to mention a few. In many studies, participant-observation as role, technique, and methodology has been of use.

Becker and Geer (1969:324) point out that participant observation coupled with an interview provides situations in which "meanings of words can be learned with great precision through study of their use in context and can also suggest something of the value system." Participant-observation makes it possible to check descriptions against fact and to identify certain "distortions" of perception that may be due to the individual's position in an organization (Becker and Geer 1969:326).

A nurse-fieldworker in a migrant health project (who concentrates on observation of the structure and function of the various clinics; outreach efforts to inform growers and workers of the services; and nurse-patient interactions during intake, screening, and referral procedures) soon begins to identify cultural, class, and role differences between client and health-care provider. Linguistic and value differences are immediately evident when one observes in the clinics. Within a reasonably short time, the observer begins to identify definitions of health and illness, including folk beliefs; family support structures; decision making directed toward seeking of health care or counseling; social networks; in the community; social functions served by the clinics for the clients, and political and economic status of the workers. Within this context the nurse participant-observer obtains a beginning understanding not only about effectiveness of the health care delivery system, but also of the patients and their health needs. Since these data come in bits and pieces, conscientious use of field notes is necessary to help sort out the information so that it can be classified and categorized into an understandable whole. Subsequently, decisions about how and where to focus research efforts can begin to be made.

Participant-Observation in Clinical Practice

Since nurses are well-versed in the inductive approach to medical and nursing diagnoses, use of participant-observation to gather information about patient's health care needs is a natural adjunct to observation of physical and behavioral symptoms in clinical nursing practice. Sharpening of observational skills and techniques to develop a more holistic picture of the patient's illness and its meaning and to check out hypotheses about patients and patient care, provides the clinical nurse with valuable data about the patient, whether it be during primary health screening or during planning and execution of short- and long-range nursing and health care.

The community health nurse is particularly fortunate in having ready access to the "natural environment" of patients and families, and in participating to varying degrees in that environment to evaluate and coordinate health-care needs. The psychosocial nurse may be an integral part of the patient's therapeutic milieu; as both participant and observer the nurse recognizes reciprocal influences in the therapist-client roles and is able to use them in working with the patient. Knowledge of subcultural beliefs, values, and practices related to maternal and child care, of family life styles, and of family membership roles, assists the nurse in helping with family planning, interpreting sexuality, coordinating and carrying out plans for care of well, ill, or handicapped children, and in the midwifery role. For the nurse caring for medical or surgical patients, knowledge of influences of the home and hospital environment on the patient's illness/wellness levels and relationship to care and cure efforts greatly enhances success of the nursing efforts.

Participant-observation can be of use to the nurse in leadership and administrative roles in a variety of health care facilities. The method can be useful in understanding organizational structure and process, formal and informal; it can help the nurse administrator develop skill in identifying significant cues to strengths and weaknesses in the organization, without screening out the "field" in which these occur. Participant-observation can reveal discrepancies between what the supervisor or administrator thinks is occurring in the organization and actual observed performances.

Evaluation as to probable receptivity to new health care programs may be assisted by participant-observation in the area where the programs are proposed. When the coordinator for a day care program for migrant workers' children states that "When this town supports something, it goes all the way," and further investigation reveals longstanding cooperation of the town's citizens on other community projects, it seems probable that if a program could be "sold" to the populace it would have a good chance of success, particularly if the people could have an active part in its operation.

When an Indian health clinic director responds to an initial question about the use of nurses in the clinic to support medical personnel by saying, "I don't want any nurse practitioners," further interview may reveal that (1) an Indian Health Service regional director had attempted to force nurse practitioners on the clinic without their consent, and (2) the clinic director believes that women could not handle combative patients as well as men. Actual observation, however, may reveal that men nurses might be acceptable or that the patients are not that difficult to handle. Decisions could be made as to whether to attempt demonstration of effectiveness of nurse practitioners through more subtle and less threatening means, with full appreciation of Indian values and beliefs.

In each of these areas of clinical and administrative practice of nursing, participant-observation as role, technique, and methodology can be a primary source of information about the broader "environment" or can be a complement to other techniques of data-gathering. As the nurse-practitioner and extended nursing roles develop more fully, it will be imperative for the professional nurse to have a method such as participant observation which can enable her/him to evaluate the total context of care for patients and its influence on their level of illness and wellness. This may, in fact, be one of the unique contributions the nurse can bring to the health care team.

SUMMARY AND FURTHER COMMENTS

The nurse participant-observer must first decide the range of participation and observation which will best yield the data needed. Second, the observer must recognize, accept, and be willing to attempt to reconcile three major dilemmas in the chosen research role: (1) objectivity and/or subjectivity, (2) scientific integrity of the study and/or protection of the rights of individuals who are subjects of the research, and (3) nonintervention and/or intervention into the activities of the study group.

Third, it is necessary to recognize the reciprocal aspects of the role as an investigator studying human subjects in the field, and to maintain an awareness of the possible effect of her/his presence on the data collected. Since this presence alone changes some of the situations studied, the ways in which the subjects view the researcher's role affects the type of feedback obtained. It would be nearly impossible to measure this effect over time, although a second observer might be able to make note of single incidents. Process-recording which includes notations of the nurse researcher's subjective reactions to specific incidents can also be useful. Data about personal feelings and attitudes serve to develop more insight into one's own behavior in the research situation; they also provide an additional check on data-gathering and analytical techniques. Such material analyzed by a qualified, but noninvolved, person, provides an additional dimension to role reciprocity and behavior. In spite of such efforts, the researcher is wise who recognizes that people's definitions of what one is and what one is doing rarely corresponds with one's own definition.

A team of researchers can make more efficient use of time and effort in a well-coordinated field study of such complex organizations as large health care facilities. Pooling of both objective data and subjective impressions from several investigators with differing disciplinary backgrounds in the same setting provides a cross-checking of data and permits discussion of various interpretations of what has been observed. Strauss, *et. al.* (1964) have demonstrated the advantages of this approach. Such a sharing of experiences is not available to the lone researcher.

While there are definite advantages in being the only investigator in the field, and being responsible alone for establishing the necessary long-term relationships with persons in the study, it is likely that a team approach could help the researcher of complex organizations to avoid some conflict of roles. This writer found it necessary to spend time with administrative personnel gathering background information on the general hospital milieu for later use in analysis of the study data. Because of this, she found herself in a type of role which made her position as observer on the nursing unit sometimes suspect to certain personnel. This situation is not unlike that of the anthropologist who must determine his relationship with authority figures in a society while maintaining the role as an investigator with the rest of the members of that society. As Wax (1971:368) warns and advises, too close an association with leaders or "people at the top" can greatly limit the scope of the fieldwork.

Longitudinal field studies present some unique problems. Not only do physical, procedural, and value changes occur in the ongoing process of day-to-day existence, for example, on a nursing unit or a rural health project, but persons present at one stage of the study may not be present during previous or subsequent stages. The presence or absence of some of these persons can be critical to the course of the study, yet it is difficult at the time to predict just who these individals may be and to what extent they affect the behavior of the total group. The end result of such a study is at once a diachronic and synchronic description of individual and patterned behavior within one unique sociocultural system; adaptive strategies and decision making in the face of continuing change can then be placed in context.

The field approach to research and to data gathering by the clinical nurse permits examination of an immediate behavioral situation in a manner that is more than purely descriptive. It permits recognition of a variety of factors which may influence the actors' choice of behavior, even though actual motivation may not be evident. Response by the nurse-investigator to the informants' handling of her/his presence can be based on perception and cognition of the complex interplay of forces operating at various levels in the setting.

In sum, the process of participant-observation involves a sensitive awareness of behaviors of the persons being observed, similar insight into the investigator's own actions and reactions, a careful and complete recording of these events, generation of hypotheses from the qualitative data, and retrospective evaluation and analysis of both hypotheses and data. The professional nurse-researcher who recognizes and makes use of the multiple facets of the participant-observer role can engage in behavioral research concerning members of the nursing profession and maintain the objectivity and integrity which such research demands. She can also make effective use of the role in collecting clinical data that enable her to make more accurate nursing diagnoses and evaluate effectiveness of patient care.

REFERENCES

Abdellah, Faye G., "Approaches to Protecting the Rights of Human Subjects," *Nursing Research* 16 (1967):316-20.

American Anthropological Association. *Professional Ethics: Statements and Procedures of the American Anthropological Association.* Washington, D. C., September 1973.

American Nurses' Association Committee on Research Studies, "The Nurse in Research: ANA Guidelines on Ethical Values," *Nursing Research* 17 (1968):104-7.

Becker, Howard, and Blanche Geer, "Participant Observation and Interviewing: A Comparison." In *Issues in Participant Observation: A Text and Reader* (McCall and Simmons, eds.). Reading, Mass.: Addison-Wesley Publishing Co., 1969, p. 324.

Becker, Howard S., "Problems of Inference and Proof in Participant Observation," *American Sociological Review* 23 (1958):652-60.

Bowen, Elenore Smith (Laura Bohannan), *Return to Laughter.* Garden City, N. Y.: Doubleday and Company Inc., Anchor Books, 1964. (First published by Harper and Brothers, 1954.)

Byerly, Elizabeth Lee, "Registered Nurse Role Behavior in the Hospital Sociocultural System: A System Approach." Unpublished doctoral dissertation, University of Washington, Department of Anthropology, Seattle, 1970.

Caudill, William, *The Psychiatric Hospital as a Small Society.* Cambridge: Harvard University Press, 1958.

Dean, John P., Robert L. Eishorn, and Louis R. Dean. "Limitations a and Advantages of Unstructured Methods." In *Issues in Participant Observation: A Text and Reader* (McCall and Simmons, eds.). Reading, Mass.: Addison-Wesley Publishing Company, 1969.

Goffman, Erving, *The Presentation of Self in Everyday Life.* New York: Doubleday and Company, Inc., Anchor Books, 1959.

Goffman, Erving, *Encounters: Two Studies in the Sociology of Interaction.* Indianapolis: The Bobbs-Merrill Company, Inc., 1961.

Kluckhohn, Florence R., "The Participant-Observer Technique in Small Communities," *The American Journal of Sociology* 46 (1940):331-343.

McCall, George J., and J. L. Simmons, eds., *Issues in Participant Observation: A Text and Reader.* Reading, Mass. Addison-Wesley Publishing Co., 1969.

Olesen, Virginia L., and Elvi W. Whittaker, *The Silent Dialogue.* San Francisco: Jossey-Bass, Inc., Publishers, 1968.

Pearsall, Marion, "Participant Observation as Role and Method in Behavioral Research," *Nursing Research* 14 (1965):37-42.

Pelto, Pertti J., *Anthropological Research: The Structure of Inquiry.* New York: Harper & Row, Publishers, 1970.

Quint, Jeanne C., "The Case for Theories Generated from Empirical Data," *Nursing Research* 16 (1967):109-14.

Read, Kenneth E., *The High Valley.* New York: Charles Scribner's Sons, 1965.

Schwartz, Morris S., and Charlotte Green Schwartz, "Problems in Participant Observation," *The American Journal of Sociology* 60 (1955):343-53.

Spiro, Melford E., *Children of the Kibbutz.* Cambridge: Harvard University Press, 1958, pp. 465-75.

Strauss, Anselm, et al., *Psychiatric Ideologies and Institutions.* New York: The Free Press of Glencoe, 1964.

Van de Bittner, Susan Kay, "An In-Depth Analysis of Health Care Delivery in Two Walk-In Clinics." Unpublished master's thesis, University of Washington, School of Nursing, Seattle, 1973, p. 26.

Vidich, Arthur J., "Participant Observation and the Collection and Interpretation of Data," *The American Journal of Sociology* 60 (1955):354-60.

Wax, Rosalie H., *Doing Fieldwork: Warnings and Advice.* Chicago: University of Chicago Press, 1971, p. 368.

Webb, Eugene J., et al., *Unobtrusive Measure: Nonreactive Research in the Social Sciences.* Chicago: Rand McNally and Company, 1966.

Whiting, Beatrice, and John Whiting, "Methods for Observing and Recording Behavior." In *A Handbook of Method in Cultural Anthropology* (Naroll and Cohen, eds.). New York: Columbia University Press, 1973.

The Ethnographic Approach and Nursing Research

ANTOINETTE T. RAGUCCI

Ragucci takes the method of participant-observation into the community. Her study of Italian-American women, across generations, provides us with a different perspective on the depth of knowledge needed by the nurse working in a community that may have one or more ethnic groups represented, or where the ethnic group is in various stages of moving toward the norms of the new (host) culture. Ragucci shows that not all Italian-American women living in an Italian-American enclave in an American city hold the same beliefs about life and health. The same findings may be elicited for other ethnic enclaves. The assessment of the degree of acculturation enhances the work of the nurse in the community.

In utilizing the ethnographic approach for the investigation of cultural phenomena related to health, the method of participant-observation, used by anthropologists to study peoples of non-Western cultures, was adapted for the investigation of cultural continuity and change in the concepts of health, curing practices, and ritual expressions of women living in an ethnic enclave of a large American city.

The focal point of the research described here centered on the discovery of "conceptual models" of health and illness of peoples who represent variants of Western and Eastern European civilization. Attention was directed toward the identification of so-called "folk" health systems, usually associated with an agrarian mode of life, as viable and functional entities within an urban milieu. The scope of interest, then, was similar to that of anthropologists who engage in research in the more recently developed areas of the science of man—medical and urban anthropology.

A concomitant interest focused upon the delineation of intra- and intercultural variations in cultural beliefs and practices about health. Most comparative studies that deal with behavioral differentials in response to illness of ethnic groups residing in American urban centers disregard or minimize the differences which may be present not only between generations but also within generations. Some studies do not specify the generational depth nor control adequately for the generation variable. A truncated sample results if the first or immigrant generation is not taken sufficiently into account. Valid generalizations about cultural differences and persistence and change in health beliefs and associated practices require adequate sampling of at least three generations, the first or foreign-born established as the base line. At present, progress in the development of a comparative frame of reference for the study of cultural differences in response to illness is impeded by the lack of descriptive data about specific subcultural groups residing in America.

Ethnographies, empirically descriptive of the real world, provide the chief analytic instruments by which valid cross-cultural comparisons are made. For example, 862 sample societies, classified in the *Ethnographic Atlas*, are sufficiently described so that they may be used for cross-cultural comparisons (Murdock, 1967). However, only 15 appear to be samples of Western or Eastern European societies.

A NATURALISTIC APPROACH

The ethnographic approach is a naturalistic comparative method aimed at studying human behavior and attitudes through observations in the natural setting. Ethnographic study or community study is a method in which "a problem or problems in the nature, interconnections or dynamics of behavior and attitudes is explored against or within the context of other behaviors and attitudes of the individuals making up the life of a particular community" (Arensberg and Kimball, 1965, p. 29). Community study is a method of observation, exploration, comparison, and verification. It is an observational rather than a statistical or experimental method.

The task of the anthropologist is to describe specific cultures adequately. The rules for the collection of cultural data using the naturalistic field research approach were explicated by Malinowski in 1922. Radcliffe-Brown (1935) and Malinowski (1922), identified with the school of functionalism, were among the first to advocate the study of cultures as functional wholes by the use of field techniques.

The basic assumption underlying the functionalist view of culture is that everything in the life of a community has a function, and what appears to be the same social usage in two or more societies may actually have different functions in each. According to Radcliffe-Brown, the acceptance of the functional hypothesis results in the recognition "of problems for the solution of which comparative studies of diverse societies and intensive study of a single society are required" (pp. 399-400).

A more recent development in ethnographic methodology is referred to as the "new ethnography" or ethnoscience. The suffix "science" is not used in the usual sense. It refers to classification or taxonomy. When used with the prefix "ethno-," ethnoscience refers to the systems of cognition typical of a given culture (Sturtevant, 1968, p. 475). Hence, ethnobotany—folk taxonomy of plants; ethnohistory—a conception of the past shared by the people of a culture; ethnomedicine—folk medical classifications or folk conceptions of phenomena associated with illness or disease.

Goodenough at a roundtable in 1957 proposed that ethnography be conceived as the discovery of the conceptual models with which a society operates. According to this view:

> A society's culture consists of whatever one has to know or believe in order to operate in a manner acceptable to its members. . . . It is the form of things that people have in mind, their models for perceiving, relating and otherwise interpreting them. . . . Ethnographic description . . . requires methods of processing observed phenomena such that we can inductively construct a theory of how our informants have organized the same pehnomena. It is the theory, not the phenomena alone, which ethnographic description aims to present (Goodenough, 1964, p. 36).

The ethnoscientific approach facilitates intracultural as well as cross-cultural comparisons. Anthropologists have borrowed the con-concepts of *etic* and *emic* as used by linguists for the study of native or folk classificatory systems. Derived from the word phonetic, etic refers to units or classifications not validated in native reactions to the behavior in question (Pike, 1964; Hymes, 1964, p. 14). Etic features are common to more than one culture, that is, they are "culture-free," and, therefore, can be utilized for cross-cultural comparative purposes. On the other hand, emic classifications are culture-bound or culture-specific. An emic approach is an attempt to "discover and describe the behavioral system of a given culture in its own terms" (French, 1963, p. 398).

The "new ethnography" raises the standards of reliability and validity in ethnography. It employs rigorous methods for the intensive study of selected cultural domains. Ethnoscience requires the specification of the discovery procedures and the validity of the descriptions depends upon the discovery procedures (Sturtevant, 1968, p. 483).

The old and new approach are not mutually exclusive. Both methods may be utilized in the same field experience. Frake (1961), for example, discovered that effective communication with the Subanun people depended upon the anthropologist's mastery of the terminology of folk medicine and botany before he could proceed to a systematic study of other cultural and structural elements.

The concept underlying ethnoscience is not a new idea. Malinowski expressed a similar view 50 years ago:

> The final goal of which the Ethnographer should never lose sight . . . is briefly to grasp the native's point of view, his relation to life, to realize *his* vision of *his* world (Malinowski, 1954, p. 25).

The size and complexity of American communities have been cited as obstacles for attaining the ethnographic ideal of studying cultures as wholes. However, the study of one aspect, for example, health, within the context of the community will allow the investigator to gain an understanding of its spatial or ecological patterns and social and cultural processes. For example, in my study (Ragucci, 1971) of the health beliefs and practices of women in an Italian-American enclave, the structure of social relationships at the level of kin, ritual kin, and neighborhood were analyzed according to the functional nature of the social links in events concerned with illness and death. In like manner, the dominant value orientations were studied according to their fit with cultural behavior during periods of crisis.

THE PARTICIPANT-OBSERVATION METHOD

A strategy was devised to insure the researcher's maximum exposure to a number of situations in which the beliefs and behaviors about health and healing were more likely to be expressed. The method of participant-observation is synonymous with the ethnographic approach. The observation process itself is part of what Nagel (1961) referred to as "controlled investigation" (p. 452).

> Scientific observation is deliberate search, carried out with care and forethought, as contrasted with the casual and largely passive perceptions of everyday life. It is this deliberateness and control of the observation process which is distinctive of science, not merely the use of special instruments (Kaplan, 1964, p. 126).

The major instrument for the collection of data is the investigator himself. Thus, the successful employment of the method of participant-observation is predicated upon one's ability to establish rapport and relationships of mutual trust and respect with his informants. The way in which the investigator defines his role may facilitate or hinder his entry into the community. For example, in collecting data for my study of the cognitive orientations and basic premises about health held by women in an Italian-American enclave, the decision about the role in which I wished to be perceived was made prior to my initial reconnaissance in the community to rent an apartment. The role had to be congruent not only with the type of research questions that I intended to ask but also with the residents' expectations of those who occupy the role. After much deliberation, I decided that the most plausible explanation for my presence in the community was that of a graduate student who was interested in studying health and the "old traditions" and customs associated with health and curing. This definition was congruent with the role I assumed for the 15-month period of residence in the enclave.

The type and location of living quarters, too, determined the quantity and quality of primary or face-to-face relationships. I rented modest living quarters in an apartment complex which had a larger number of units than the typical tenement. After moving into the community, I discovered my decision had been a fortunate one. Rental of a cold water flat, one of the choices, would have lowered my status with my neighbors. On the other hand, occupancy of a remodeled luxury-type apartment rented to middle-class professionals considered "outsiders" by the older residents would have increased social distance.

The time table and circumstances relative to entry in the social world of the women varied according to generation. Four months elapsed before I was accepted as a neighbor and friend. Some factors which facilitated acceptance by the women in the oldest age class, the established base line group, were my identity as a second-generation

Italian who could communicate in the native tongue and the ascription of the role of "literati" by those women who lacked literary and language skills in English. The strategy of using the quotations of Italian proverbs, the repositories of folk wisdom, was particularly effective in establishing rapport with women who were initially resistant to the researcher's attempts to elicit information about their traditional and contemporary customs and beliefs. This resistance might be viewed from the perspective of women who probably were sensitive to the criticism of their children for holding "superstitious" ideas.

Status differentials delayed entry into the social world of second-generation women. The problems associated with social distance decreased as I immersed myself in neighborhood and community activities. The establishment of a symmetrical dyadic relationship with a neighbor was probably the most important single factor for my eventual acceptance within the established neighborhood social structure. In the community, the principle which defined the social relationships of the first- and older second-generation women, for example, those above 50 years of age, was that derived from the model of the dyadic contract. According to Foster (1961), this model is consistent with the form of interpersonal relationships which prevail in some European Mediterranean peasant societies. Reciprocity is the basic integrative principle of the implicit dyadic contract which serves to link a person to certain relatives, neighbors, or friends to the exclusion of others who occupy the same status (Foster, p. 1174).

Age differentials limited participation in the social activities of the women of the third generation. To counteract this, data were collected by means of unstructured interviews and unobtrusive observations of mothers who brought their children to the weekly well-child conference. At this time I had the opportunity to check out observations made in my interactions with the older women during the week. Contact with these women continued through the period of time required for the completion of their children's immunization program. Casual meetings in neighborhood stores and markets and at social functions provided additional contacts.

Primary relationships were established with ten first-generation women, 12 second-generation, and three in the youngest age group. These women, in turn, introduced me to a wider circle of their relatives and friends who resided in different sectors of the enclave.

Small Group Structure. The anthropological ideal of collecting data within the context of the natural setting was accomplished mainly through the medium of the small group structure prevalent in the enclave. During the summer months we sat in front of the tenement, and in the winter we moved to the warmth of the kitchen. Current ailments, deaths, or hospitalization of neighbors and friends would invariably appear as topics for discussion. Some visits were specifically oriented to fulfill one's obligations to the sick and ailing. The neighbors customarily gathered at the homes of hospitalized persons when family members returned from the afternoon or evening hospital visiting hours. A veritable mine of data was collected on these occasions. The family members would report their perceptions of the progress of the hospitalized person, the perceived rationale of the prescribed treatment and, very often, their perception of the quality of medical and nursing care administered to the relative.

In the later phase of field work, efforts were directed toward reaching women who were marginal to the established neighborhood social systems. These women, many of whom were economically marginal, were dependent upon various formal community organizations for meeting their social and recreational needs. Data were collected by means of informal interviews during the social hours which followed the regular programs.

A retired visiting nurse, who had ministered to the health needs of the enclave for over 30 years, was instrumental in introducing me to women emigrants of a region in Italy whose folklore of health and healing had been documented at the turn of the century (Pitre, 1871-1913, 1896). This provided the opportunity to assess the persistence and change in beliefs and practices of this variant group utilizing an historical source for base line information.

Unobtrusive observations at such diverse social occasions as wakes and picnics yielded a wealth of pertinent data. Wakes provide a setting where folk or laymen's theories about the etiology of disease and cause of death are more likely to be expressed. An opportunity to assess the current usages of herbal remedies by members of the first and second generation occurred during a combined picnic and pilgrimage to a religious shrine located in a rural area. Elderly women used this occasion to replenish their supply of herbs, and the researcher was able to elicit the people's beliefs about the curing properties of these substances. On the other hand, unobtrusive observations at the local pharmacies enabled the researcher to determine current usages of patent medicines. By means of unstructured interviews, additional data about the layman's use of pharmaceutical preparations were obtained from the pharmacists.

Data Classification. The data collected by means of this essentially qualitative inductive approach were organized and recorded in several ways. Field notes, life histories, and a personal diary constituted the chief records of the field research; 35 mm. slides of the public events and rituals associated with the patron saint societies were made. Data were processed according to the categories listed in *The Outline of Cultural Materials* (Murdock *et al.*, 1967), a tool developed for the Cross-Cultural Survey at the Institute for Human Relations at Yale University.

A typology, "Traditional Folk Medicine" and "Contemporary Folk Medicine," was constructed to serve as a heuristic device for the organization and analysis of data along the generational dimension. The theoretical bases for the typology were: Redfield's (1947) construct of the folk-urban continuum and his concepts of the "great" and "little" traditions; Ackerknecht's (1942, 1946) theories on the nature of primitive and folk medicine; Levi-Strauss' (1966) "Science of the Concrete"; and Freidson's (1961) differentiation of modern medical and layman's knowledge. The users of "Traditional Folk Medicine" focus upon the concrete qualitative aspects of the substances employed for cure or prevention of illness. This type exhibits correspondingly more features embedded in a magical-religious frame of reference than the contemporary. The pharmacopoeia consists mainly of elements found in nature. Cultural or medical lag is revealed by the presence of traits similar to those held by older medical traditions, i.e., Greek-Roman or early twentieth-century medicine.

"Contemporary Folk Medicine" consists of elements which have filtered down from modern medicine and which have been reinterpreted by the layman. Magical-religious conceptualizations do not occupy a prominent role in the curing system, and the pharmacopoeia consists largely of manufactured or patent remedies.

The accumulating field record was reviewed at frequent, usually daily, intervals. The regularly recurring behaviors or events were noted, and patterns or configurations were isolated. Tentative or working hypotheses were formulated as guides for future inquiry. Significant events and interactions were recorded according to two categories, "act meaning" and "action meaning." As used here, "act meaning" refers to the people's explanation or definition of an event or behavior, that is, the semantic explanation. "Action meaning" refers to the meaning of the event or behavior from the perspective of the investigator, that is, the theoretical explanation of the event (see Kaplan, 1964, pp. 358-363).

The personal diary functioned as a "dialogue with self." It provided a means by which observations were insulated by focusing attention upon those factors which might have interferred with the achievement of the necessary detachment or objectivity. Most notations dealt with problems associated with value conflicts between those being observed and the observer, overidentification with the group, doubts about the ethical validity of collecting data by means of an essentially indirect and unobtrusive method, and conflicts relative to the exploitation of relationships as means to an end not always fully understood by my informants. One of the most problematic issues was the role conflict engendered by the constraints imposed upon a health professional when incorrect or irrelevant health beliefs or practices were noted. Deliberate and planned intervention occurred when the occasion demanded it, that is, when a belief or practice was known to be potentially or actually harmful.

These records of field research provide the raw materials from which data are selected for the ethnography. A qualitative inductive method of data collection presents a formidable challenge for the organization of the final account. The task of separating interpretations from descriptions is difficult, and the report of findings does not always yield elegant explanations.

USES FOR ETHNOGRAPHY

However, the advantages in the use of this method outweigh its costs. The ethnographic approach is most effective for the study of groups whose members do not have the literary and language skills characteristic of the dominant white middle-class culture. The method of participant-observation permits entry into cultures which would otherwise be inaccessible by reason of their marginality or style of life. For example, the child psychiatrist, Robert Coles (1970), adapted the methods of the social anthropologist for the study of the early life of migrant workers. The method of participant-observation allows the investigator to look beyond reports of behavior and to observe the behavior itself so that he can assess the correspondence or the discrepancy that exists between the real and the ideal cultural statements. Finally, prolonged residence in a community and the continuing relationships provide more opportunity to check the reliability of informants.

The ethnographic study of urban communities will probably best be accomplished by means of the coordinated efforts of a research team. In the division of labor within the fields of medical and urban anthropology, the basic task of the nurse-anthropologist appears to be that of the ethnographer of the "health cultures" of the various subcultural groups which make up the population of large urban centers.

The investigation of the functional relationships and the interconnections of health, social structure, and culture need not be restricted to the community. Ethnographies of the natural settings in which behaviors and attitudes related to health and illness are more likely to be expressed—namely, the hospital, the clinical division, the health center, or the nursing home—need to be compiled. The ethnography of these samples of social and cultural systems should be written from the point of view of the people who are recipients of health services.

An alternate approach, the ethnoscientific, will enable the nurse-ethnographer to describe adequately the phenomena associated with health and illness according to the conceptual systems of the people she is studying. Having identified a culture's or a patient's model for perceiving, relating, or otherwise interpreting health phenomena, she can inductively construct a theory of how her informants or patients have organized the same phenomena (see Goodenough, 1964).

The ethnoscientific method is most effectively used within the context of the natural setting. In the study of the women residents of an ethnic enclave, I constructed theories of how people perceived health and illness by listening to their conversations and eliciting information within the context of situations specifically oriented to illness experiences.

An interesting area of ethnoscientific exploration is ethnophysiology, a domain which refers to the classification of human physiology by the folk or laymen. Because I hold an appointment as associate in nursing, I can explore this area while engaging in the administration of nursing care on the medical-surgical clinical division. The ultimate objective is to devise a method which can be replicated for the study of intracultural and intercultural similarities and differences in the classification of the same phenomena. The use of a three-generation design in this area may pose formidable problems in eliciting information from non-English-speaking people because the introduction of a translator will change the natural research setting. A more immediate problem concerns the framing of the research questions. Therefore, I am currently concentrating on the task of phrasing the eliciting questions without the imposition of my own preconceived categories of human physiology.

The ethnographic is an appropriate methodological approach to the study of the cognitive and affective orientations of diverse urban subcultural groups and the mode of their responses to the processes of acculturation considered within the perspective of health and medical systems. It has a place in nursing science. For, the final goal—of which the nurse-ethnographer should never lose sight—is to grasp the patient's point of view, his relations to life, to realize his vision of the phenomena of health and illness.

REFERENCES

Ackerknecht, E. H. Problems of primitive medicine. *Bull. Hist. Med.* 11:503-521, May 1942.

_____. Natural disease and rational treatment in primitive medicine. *Bull. Hist. Med.* 19:467-497, May 1946.

Arensberg, C. M., and Kimball, S. T. *Culture and Community.* New York, Harcourt, Brace and World, 1965.

Coles, Robert. *Uprooted Children.* New York, Harper and Row Publishers, 1970.

Foster, G. M. What is folk culture? *Am. Anthropologist* 55:159-173, Apr.-June 1953.

_____. The dyadic contract: a model for the social structure of a Mexican peasant village. *Am. Anthropologist* 63:1173-1192, Dec. 1961.

Frake, C. O. Diagnosis of disease among Subanun of Mindanao. *Am. Anthropologist* 63:113-132, Feb. 1961.

Freidson, Eliot. *Patients' Views of Medical Practice.* New York, Russell Sage Foundation, 1961.

French, David. The relationship of anthropology to studies in perception and cognition. In *Psychology; a Study of a Science,* edited by Sigmund Koch. New York, McGraw-Hill Book Co., 1963, Vol. 6, pp. 388-428.

Gans, Herbert. *The Urban Villagers.* New York, Free Press, 1962.

Goodenough, W. H. Cultural anthropology and linguistics. In *Language in Culture and Society,* edited by Dell Hymes. New York, Harper and Row, 1964, pp. 36-39.

Hymes, Dell, ed. *Language in Culture and Society.* New York, Harper and Row, 1964.

Kaplan, Abraham. *The Conduct of Inquiry.* San Francisco, Chandler Publishing Co., 1964.

Lévi-Strauss, Claude. *The Savage Mind.* London, Wiedenfeld and Nicholson, 1966.

Malinowski, Bronislaw. *Argonauts of the Western Pacific.* Prospect Heights, IL: Waveland Press, Inc., 1984. (Orginally published in 1922).

Murdock, G. P. *Ethnographic Atlas.* Pittsburgh, University of Pittsburgh Press, 1967.

_____ and others. *Outline of Cultural Materials.* New Haven, Human Relations Area File, 1967.

Nagel, Ernest. The Structure of Science. New York, Harcourt, Brace and World, 1961.

Pike, Kenneth. Toward a theory of the structure of human behavior. In *Language in Culture and Society,* edited by Dell Hymes. New York, Harper and Row, 1964, pp. 54-62.

Pitrè, Giuseppe. *Biblioteca delle Tradizione Popolare Siciliane.* 25 Volumes, Palermo, Italy, L. Pedone-Lauriel di Carlo Clausen, 1871-1913.

_____. *Medicina Popolare Siciliana.* Torino-Palermo, Italy, L. Pedone-Lauriel di Carlo Clausen, 1896.

Radcliffe-Brown, A. R. On the concept of function in social science. *Am. Anthropologist* 37:394-402, July-Sept. 1935.

Ragucci, A. T. *Generational Continuity and Change in the Concepts of Health, Curing Practices and Ritual Expressions of the Women of an Italian-American Enclave.* Boston, Mass., Boston University, 1971. (Unpublished Ph.D. dissertation)

Redfield, Robert. The folk society. *Am. J. Sociol.* 52:293-308, Jan. 1947.

Sturtevant, W. C. Studies in ethnoscience. In *Theory in Anthropology,* edited by Robert A. Manners and David Kaplan. Chicago, Aldine Publishing Co., 1968, pp. 475-500.

On Being Sane in Insane Places

D.L. ROSENHAN

Rosenhan describes the methods of participant-observation from the perspective of the health care consumer. As can be seen, role taking in regard to the patient role is not particularly difficult. Although this article is highly entertaining, several points must be kept in mind. First, the patient's perspective of the health care delivery system is not necessarily complimentary. Second, psychiatry, unlike other fields of medicine, frequently accepts the patient's valuation of himself as ill until further determination of disease process can be made. Third, health professionals interact with the label patient and not with patients as individuals. Last, as a research method, participant observation is not believed to be an objective or scientific research method, as can be seen from the furor raised by this article. (See Science, April 27, 1973)

If sanity and insanity exist, how shall we know them?

The question is neither capricious nor itself insane. However much we may be personally convinced that we can tell the normal from the abnormal, the evidence is simply not compelling. It is commonplace, for example, to read about murder trials wherein eminent psychiatrists for the defense are contradicted by equally eminent psychiatrists for the prosecution on the matter of the defendant's sanity. More generally, there are a great deal of conflicting data on the reliability, utility, and meaning of such terms as "sanity," "insanity," "mental illness," and "schizophrenia" (*1*). Finally, as early as 1934, Benedict suggested that normality and abnormality are not universal (*2*). What is viewed as normal in one culture may be seen as quite abberrant in another. Thus, notions of normality and abnormality may not be quite as accurate as people believe they are.

To raise questions regarding normality and abnormality is in no way to question the fact that some behaviors are deviant or odd. Murder is deviant. So, too, are hallucinations. Nor does raising such questions deny the existence of the personal anguish that is often associated with "mental illness." Anxiety and depression exist. Psychological suffering exists. But normality and abnormality, sanity and insanity, and the diagnoses that flow from them may be less substantive than many believe them to be.

At its heart, the question of whether the sane can be distinguished from the insane (and whether degrees of insanity can be distinguished from each other) is a simple matter: do the salient characteristics that lead to diagnoses reside in the patients themselves or in the environments and contexts in which observers find them? From Bleuler, through Kretchmer, through the formulators of the recently revised *Diagnostic and Statistical Manual* of the American Psychiatric Association, the belief has been strong that patients present symptoms, that those symptoms can be categorized, and, implicitly, that the sane are distinguishable from the insane. More recently, however, this belief has been questioned. Based in part on theoretical and anthropological considerations, but also on philosophical, legal, and therapeutic ones, the view has grown that psychological categorization of mental illness is useless at best and downright harmful, misleading, and pejorative at worst. Psychiatric diagnoses, in this view, are in the minds of the observers and are not valid summaries of characteristics displayed by the observed (*3-5*).

Gains can be made in deciding which of these is more nearly accurate by getting normal people (that is, people who do not have, and have never suffered, symptoms of serious psychiatric disorders) admitted to psychiatric hospitals and then determining whether they were discovered to be sane and, if so, how. If the sanity of such pseudopatients were always detected, there would be prima facie evidence that a sane individual can be distinguished from the insane context in which he is found. Normality (and presumably abnormality) is distinct enough that it can be recognized wherever it occurs, for it is carried within the person. If, on the other hand, the sanity of the pseudopatients were never discovered, serious difficulties would arise for those who support traditional modes of psychiatric diagnosis. Given that the hospital staff was not incompetent, that the pseudopatient had been behaving as sanely as he had been outside of the hospital, and that it had never been previously suggested that he belonged in a psychiatric hospital, such an unlikely outcome would support the view that psychiatric diagnosis betrays little about the patient but much about the environment in which an observer finds him.

This article describes such an experiment. Eight sane people gained secret admission to 12 different hospitals (*6*). Their diagnostic experiences constitute the data of the first part of this article; the remainder is devoted to a description of their experiences in psychiatric institutions. Too few psychiatrists and psychologists, even those who have worked in such hospitals, know what the experience is like. They rarely talk about it with former patients, perhaps because they distrust information coming from the previously insane. Those who have worked in psychiatric hospitals are likely to have adapted so thoroughly to the settings that they are insensitive to the impact of that experience. And while there have been occasional reports of researchers who submitted themselves to psychiatric hospitalization (*7*), these researchers have commonly remained in the hospitals for short periods of time, often with the knowledge of the hospital staff. It is difficult to know the extent to which they were treated like patients or like research colleagues. Nevertheless, their reports about the inside of the psychiatric hospital have been valuable. This article extends those efforts.

PSEUDOPATIENTS AND THEIR SETTINGS

The eight pseudopatients were a varied group. One was a psychology graduate student in his 20's. The remaining seven were older and "established." Among them were three psychologists, a pediatrician, a psychiatrist, a painter, and a housewife. Three pseudopatients were women, five were men. All of them employed pseudonyms, lest their alleged diagnoses embarrass them later. Those who were in mental health professions alleged another occupation in order to avoid the special attentions that might be accorded by staff, as a matter of courtesy or caution, to ailing colleagues (*8*). With the exception of myself (I was the first pseudopatient and my presence was known to the hospital administrator and chief psychologist and, so far as I can tell, to them alone), the presence of pseudopatients and the nature of the research program was not known to the hospital staffs (*9*).

The settings were similarly varied. In order to generalize the findings, admission into a variety of hospitals was sought. The 12 hospitals in the sample were located in five different states on the East and West coasts. Some were old and shabby, some were quite new. Some were research-oriented, others not. Some had good staff-patient ratios, others were quite understaffed. Only one was a strictly private hospital. All of the others were supported by state or federal funds or, in one instance, by university funds.

After calling the hospital for an appointment, the peudeopatient arrived at the admission office complaining that he had been hearing voices. Asked what the voices said, he replied that they were often unclear, but as far as he could tell they said "empty," "hollow," and "thud." The voices were unfamiliar and were of the same sex as the pseudopatient. The choice of these symptoms was occasioned by their apparent similarity to existential symptoms. Such symptoms are alleged to arise from painful concerns about the perceived meaninglessness of one's life. It is as if the hallucinating person were saying, "My life is empty and hollow." The choice of these symptoms was also determined by the *absence* of a single report of existential psychoses in the literature.

Beyond alleging the symptoms and falsifying name, vocation, and employment, no further alterations of person, history, or circumstances were made. The significant events of the pseudopatient's life history were presented as they had actually occurred. Relationships with parents and siblings, with spouse and children, with people at work and in school, consistent with the aforementioned exceptions, were described as they were or had been. Frustrations and upsets were described along with joys and satisfactions. These facts are important to remember. If anything, they strongly biased the subsequent results in favor of detecting sanity, since none of their histories or current behaviors were seriously pathological in any way.

Immediately upon admission to the psychiatric ward, the pseudopatient ceased simulating *any* symptoms of abnormality. In some cases, there was a brief period of mild nervousness and anxiety, since none of the pseudopatients really believed that they would be admitted so easily. Indeed, their shared fear was that they would be immediately exposed as frauds and greatly embarrassed. Moreover, many of them had never visited a psychiatric ward; even those who had, nevertheless had some genuine fears about what might happen to them. Their nervousness, then, was quite appropriate to the novelty of the hospital setting, and it abated rapidly.

Apart from that short-lived nervousness, the pseudopatient behaved on the ward as he "normally" behaved. The pseudopatient spoke to patients and staff as he might ordinarily. Because there is uncommonly little to do on a psychiatric ward, he attempted to engage others in conversation. When asked by staff how he was feeling, he indicated that he was fine, that he no longer experienced symptoms. He responded to instructions from attendants, to calls for medication (which was not swallowed), and to dining-hall instructions. Beyond such activities as were available to him on the admissions ward, he spent his time writing down his observations about the ward, its patients, and the staff. Initially these notes were written "secretly," but as it soon became clear that no one much cared, they were subsequently written on standard tablets of paper in such public places as the dayroom. No secret was made of these activities.

The pseudopatient, very much as a true psychiatric patient, entered a hospital with no foreknowledge of when he would be discharged. Each was told that he would have to get out by his own devices, essentially by convincing the staff that he was sane. The psychological stresses associated with hospitalization were considerable, and all but one of the pseudopatients desired to be discharged almost immediately after being admitted. They were, therefore, motivated not only to behave sanely, but to be paragons of cooperation. That their behavior was in no way disruptive is confirmed by nursing reports, which have been obtained on most of the patients. These reports uniformly indicate that the patients were "friendly," "cooperative," and "exhibited no abnormal indications."

THE NORMAL ARE NOT DETECTABLY SANE

Despite their public "show" of sanity, the pseudopatients were never detected. Admitted, except in one case, with a diagnosis of schizophrenia (*10*), each was discharged with a diagnosis of schizophrenia "in remission." The label "in remission" should in no way be dismissed as a formality, for at no time during any hospitalization had any question been raised about any pseudopatient's simulation. Nor are there any indications in the hospital records that the pseudopatient's status was suspect. Rather, the evidence is strong that, once labeled schizophrenic, the pseudopatient was stuck with that label. If the pseudopatient was to be discharged, he must naturally be "in remission"; but he was not sane, nor, in the institution's view, had he ever been sane.

The uniform failure to recognize sanity cannot be attributed to the quality of the hospitals, for, although there were considerable variations among them, several are considered excellent. Nor can it be alleged that there was simply not enough time to observe the pseudopatients. Length of hospitalization ranged from 7 to 52 days, with an average of 19 days. The pseudopatients were not, in fact, carefully observed, but this failure clearly speaks more to traditions within psychiatric hospitals than to lack of opportunity.

Finally, it cannot be said that the failure to recognize the pseudopatients' sanity was due to the fact that they were not behaving sanely. While there was clearly some tension present in all of them, their daily visitors could detect no serious behavioral consequences— nor, indeed, could other patients. It was quite common for the patients to "detect" the pseudopatients' sanity. During the first three hospitalizations, when accurate counts were kept, 35 of a total of 118 patients on the admissions ward voiced their suspicions, some vigorously. "Your vigorously. You're a journalist, or a professor [referring to the continual note-taking]. You're checking up on the hospital." While most of the patients were reassured by the pseudopatient's insistence that he had been sick before he came in but was fine now, some continued to believe that the pseudopatient was sane throughout his hospitalization (*11*). The fact that the patients often recognized normality when staff did not raises important questions.

Failure to detect sanity during the course of hospitalization may be due to the fact that physicians operate with a strong bias toward what statisticians call the type 2 error (*5*). This is to say that physicians are more inclined to call a healthy person sick (a false positive, type 2) than a sick person healthy (a false negative, type 1). The reasons for this are not hard to find: it is clearly more dangerous to misdiagnose illness than health. Better to err on the side of caution, to suspect illness even among the healthy.

But what holds for medicine does not hold equally well for psychiatry. Medical illnesses, while unfortunate, are not commonly pejorative. Psychiatric diagnoses, on the contrary, carry with them personal, legal, and social stigmas (*12*). It was therefore important to see whether the tendency toward diagnosing the sane insane could be reversed. The following experiment was arranged at a research and teaching hospital whose staff had heard these findings but doubted that such an error could occur in their hospital. The staff was informed that at some time during the following 3 months, one or more pseudopatients would attempt to be admitted into the psychiatric hospital. Each staff member was asked to rate each patient who presented himself at admissions or on the ward according to the likelihood that the patient was a pseudopatient. A 10-point scale was used, with a 1 and 2 reflecting high confidence that the patient was a psudopatient.

Judgments were obtained on 193 patients who were admitted for psychiatric treatment. All staff who had had sustained contact with or primary responsibility for the patient—attendants, nurses, psychiatrists, physicians, and psychologists—were asked to make judgments. Forty-one patients were alleged, with high confidence, to be pseudopatients by at least one member of the staff. Twenty-three were considered suspect by at least one psychiatrist. Nineteen were suspected by one psychiatrist *and* one other staff member. Actually, no genuine pseudopatient (at least from my group) presented himself during this time period.

The experiment is instructive. It indicates that the tendency to designate sane people as insane can be reversed when the stakes (in this case, prestige and diagnostic acumen) are high. But what can be said of the 19 people who were suspected of being "sane" by one psychiatrist and another staff member? Were these people truly "sane," or was it rather the case that in the course of avoiding the type 2 error the staff tended to make more errors of the first sort —calling the crazy "sane"? There is no way of knowing. But one thing is certain: any diagnostic process that lends itself so readily to massive errors of this sort cannot be a very reliable one.

THE STICKINESS OF PSYCHODIAGNOSTIC LABELS

Beyond the tendency to call the healthy sick—a tendency that accounts better for diagnostic behavior on admission than it does for such behavior after a lengthy period of exposure—the data speak to the massive role of labeling in psychiatric assessment. Having once been labeled schizophrenic, there is nothing the pseudopateint can do to overcome the tag. The tag profoundly colors others' perceptions of him and his behavior.

From one viewpoint, these data are hardly surprising, for it has long been known that elements are given meaning by the context in which they occur. Gestalt psychology made this point vigorously, and Asch (*13*) demonstrated that there are "central" personality traits (such as "warm" versus "cold") which are so powerful that they markedly color the meaning of other information in forming an impression of a given personality (*14*). "Insane," "schizophrenic," "manic-depressive," and "crazy" are probably among the most powerful of such central traits. Once a person is designated abnormal, all of his other behaviors and characteristics are colored by that label. Indeed, that label is so powerful that many of the pseudopatients' normal behaviors were overlooked entirely or profoundly misinterpreted. Some examples may clarify this issue.

Earlier I indicated that there were no changes in the pseudopatients' personal history and current status beyond those of name, employment, and where necessary, vocation. Otherwise, a veridical description of personal history and circumstances was offered. Those circumstances were not psychotic. How were they made consonant with the diagnosis of psychosis? Or were those diagnoses modified in such a way as to bring them into accord with the circumstances of the pseudopatient's life, as described by him?

As far as I can determine, diagnoses were in no way affected by the relative health of the circumstances of a pseudopatient's life. Rather, the reverse occurred: the perception of his circumstances was shaped entirely by the diagnosis. A clear example of such translation is found in the case of a pseudopatient who had had a close relationship with his mother but was rather remote from his father during his early childhood. During adolescence and beyond, however, his father became a close friend, while his relationship with his mother cooled. His present relationship with his wife was characteristically close and warm. Apart from occasional angry exchanges, friction was minimal. The children had rarely been spanked. Surely there is nothing especially pathological about such a history. Indeed, many readers may see a similar pattern in their own experiences, with no markedly deleterious consequences. Observe, however, how such a history was translated in the psychopathological context, this from the case summary prepared after the patient was discharged.

> This white 39-year-old male . . . manifests a long history of considerable ambivalence in close relationships, which begins in early childhood. A warm relationship with his mother cools during his adolescence. A distant relationship to his father is described as becoming very intense. Affective stability is absent. His attempts to control emotionality with his wife and children are punctuated by angry outbursts and, in the case of the children, spankings. And while he says that he has several good friends, one senses considerable ambivalence embedded in those relationships also. . . .

The facts of the case were unintentionally distorted by the staff to achieve consistency with a popular theory of the dynamics of a schizophrenic reaction (*15*). Nothing of an ambivalent nature had been described in relations with parents, spouse, or friends. To the extent that ambivalence could be inferred, it was probably not greater than is found in all human relationships. It is true the pseudopatient's relationships with his parents changed over time, but in the ordinary context that would hardly be remarkable—indeed, it might very well be expected. Clearly, the meaning ascribed to his verbalizations (that is, ambivalence, affective instability) was determined by the diagnosis: schizophrenia. An entirely different meaning would have been ascribed if it were known that the man was "normal."

All pseudopatients took extensive notes publicly. Under ordinary circumstances, such behavior would have raised questions in the minds of observers, as, in fact, it did among patients. Indeed, it seemed so certain that the notes would elicit suspicion that elaborate precautions were taken to remove them from the ward each day. But the precautions proved needless. The closest any staff member came to questioning these notes occurred when one pseudopatient asked his physician what kind of medication he was receiving and began to write down the response. "You needn't write it," he was told gently. "If you have trouble remembering, just ask me again."

If no questions were asked of the pseudopatients, how was their writing interpreted? Nursing records for three patients indicate that the writing was seen as an aspect of their pathological behavior. "Patient engages in writing behavior" was the daily nursing comment on one of the pseudopatients who was never questioned about his writing. Given that the patient is in the hospital, he must be psychologically disturbed. And given that he is disturbed, continuous writing must be a behavioral manifestation of that disturbance, perhaps a subset of the compulsive behaviors that are sometimes correlated with schizophrenia.

One tacit characteristic of psychiatric diagnosis is that it locates the sources of aberration within the individual and only rarely within the complex of stimuli that surrounds him. Consequently, behaviors that are stimulated by the environment are commonly misattributed to the patient's disorder. For example, one kindly nurse found a pseudopatient pacing the long hospital corridors. "Nervous, Mr. X?" she asked. "No, bored," he said.

The notes kept by pseudopatients are full of patient behaviors that were misinterpreted by well-intentioned staff. Often enough, a patient would go "berserk" because he had, wittingly or unwittingly, been mistreated by, say, an attendant. A nurse coming upon the scene would rarely inquire even cursorily into the environmental stimuli of the patient's behavior. Rather, she assumed that his upset derived from his pathology, not from his present interactions with other staff members. Occasionally, the staff might assume that the patient's family (especially when they had recently visited) or other patients had stimulated the outburst. But never were the staff found to assume that one of themselves or the structure of the hospital had anything to do with a patient's behavior. One psychiatrist pointed to a group of patients who were sitting outside the cafeteria entrance half an hour before lunchtime. To a group of young residents he indicated that such behavior was characteristic of the oral-acquisitive nature of the syndrome. It seemed not to occur to him that there were very few things to anticipate in a psychiatric hospital besides eating.

A psychiatric label has a life and an influence of its own. Once the impression has been formed that the patient is schizophrenic, the expectation is that he will continue to be schizophrenic. When a sufficient amount of time has passed, during which the patient has done nothing bizarre, he is considered to be in remission and available for discharge. But the label endures beyond discharge, with the unconfirmed expectation that he will behave as a schizophrenic again. Such labels, conferred by mental health professionals, are as influential on the patient as they are on his relatives and friends, and it should not surprise anyone that the diagnosis acts on all of them as a self-fulfilling prophecy. Eventually, the patient himself accepts the diagnosis, with all of its surplus meanings and expectations, and behaves accordingly (*5*).

The inferences to be made from these matters are quite simple. Much as Zigler and Phillips have demonstrated that there is enormous overlap in the symptoms presented by patients who have been variously diagnosed (*16*), so there is enormous overlap in the behaviors of the sane and the insane. The sane are not "sane" all of the time. We lose our tempers "for no good reason." We are occasionally depressed or anxious, again for no good reason. And we may find it difficult to get along with one or another person—again for no reason that we can specify. Similarly, the insane are not always insane. Indeed, it was the impression of the pseudopatients while living with them that they were sane for long periods of time—that the bizarre behaviors upon which their diagnoses were allegedly predicated constituted only a small fraction of their total behavior. If it makes no sense to label ourselves permanently depressed on the basis of an occasional depression, then it takes better evidence than is presently available to label all patients insane or schizophrenic on the basis of bizarre behaviors or cognitions. It seems more useful, as Mischel (*17*) has pointed out, to limit our discussions to *behaviors*, the stimuli that provoke them, and their correlates.

It is not known why powerful impressions of personality traits, such as "crazy" or "insane," arise. Conceivably, when the origins of and stimuli that give rise to a behavior are remote or unknown, or when the behavior strikes us as immutable, trait labels regarding the *behaver* arise. When, on the other hand, the origins and stimuli are known and available, discourse is limited to the behavior itself. Thus, I may hallucinate because I am sleeping, or I may hallucinate because I have ingested a peculiar drug. These are termed sleep-induced hallucinations, or dreams, and drug-induced hallucinations, respectively. But when the stimuli to my hallucinations are unknown, that is called craziness, or schizophrenia—as if that inference were somehow as illuminating as the others.

THE EXPERIENCE OF PSYCHIATRIC HOSPITALIZATION

The term "mental Illness" is of recent origin. It was coined by people who were humane in their inclinations and who wanted very much to raise the station of (and the public's sympathies toward) the psychologically disturbed from that of witches and "crazies" to one that was akin to the physically ill. And they were at least partially successful, for the treatment of the mentally ill *has* improved considerably over the years. But while treatment has improved, it is doubtful that people really regard the mentally ill in the same way that they view the physically ill. A broken leg is something one recovers from, but mental illness allegedly endures forever (*18*). A broken leg does not threaten the observer, but a crazy schizophrenic? There is by now a host of evidence that attitudes toward the mentally ill are characterized by fear, hostility, aloofness, suspicion, and dread (*19*). The mentally ill are society's lepers.

That such attitudes infect the general population is perhaps not surprising, only upsetting. But that they affect the professionals—attendants, nurses, physicians, psychologists, and social workers—who treat and deal with the mentally ill is more disconcerting, both because such attitudes are self-evidently pernicious and because they are unwitting. Most mental health professionals would insist that they are sympathetic toward the mentally ill, that they are neither avoidant nor hostile. But it is more likely that an exquisite ambivalence characterizes their relations with psychiatric patients, such that their avowed impulses are only part of their entire attitude. Negative attitudes are there too and can easily be detected. Such attitudes should not surprise us. They are the natural offspring of the labels patients wear and the places in which they are found.

Consider the structure of the typical psychiatric hospital. Staff and patients are strictly segregated. Staff have their own living space, including their dining facilities, bathrooms, and assembly places. The glassed quarters that contain the professional staff, which the pseudopatients came to call "the cage," sit out on every dayroom. The staff emerge primarily for caretaking purposes—to give medication, to conduct a therapy or group meeting, to instruct or reprimand a patient. Otherwise, staff keep to themselves, almost as if the disorder that afflicts their charges is somehow catching.

So much is a patient-staff segregation the rule that, for four public hospitals in which an attempt was made to measure the degree to which staff and patients mingle, it was necessary to use "time out of the staff cage" as the operational measure. While it was not the case that all time spent out of the cage was spent mingling with patients (attendants, for example, would occasionally emerge to watch television in the dayroom), it was the only way in which one could gather reliable data on time for measuring.

The average amount of time spent by attendants outside of the cage was 11.3 percent (range, 3 to 52 percent). This figure does not represent only time spent mingling with patients, but also includes time spent on such chores as folding laundry, supervising patients while they shave, directing ward cleanup, and sending patients to off-ward activities. It was the relatively rare attendant who spent time talking with patients or playing games with them. It proved impossible to obtain a "percent mingling time" for nurses, since the amount of time they spent out of the cage was too brief. Rather, we counted instances of emergence from the cage. On the average, daytime nurses emerged from the cage 11.5 times per shift, including instances when they left the ward entirely (range, 4 to 39 times). Late afternoon and night nurses were even less available, emerging on the average 9.4 times per shift (range, 4 to 41 times). Data on early morning nurses, who arrived usually after midnight and departed at 8 a.m., are not available because patients were asleep during most of this period.

Physicians, especially psychiatrists, were even less available. They were rarely seen on the wards. Quite commonly, they would be seen only when they arrived and departed, with the remaining time being spent in their offices or in the cage. On the average, physicians emerged on the ward 6.7 times per day (range, 1 to 17 times). It proved difficult to make an accurate estimate in this regard, since physicians often maintained hours that allowed them to come and go at different times.

The hierarchical organization of the psychiatric hospital has been commented on before (*20*), but the latent meaning of that kind of organization is worth noting again. Those with the most power have least to do with patients, and those with the least power are most involved with them. Recall, however, that the acquisition of role-appropriate behaviors occurs mainly through the observation of others, with the most powerful having the most influence. Consequently, it is understandable that attendants not only spend more time with patients than do any other members of the staff—that is required by their station in the hierarchy—but also, insofar as they learn from their superiors' behavior, spend as little time with patients as they can. Attendants are seen mainly in the cage, which is where the models, the action, and the power are.

I turn now to a different set of studies, these dealing with staff response to patient-initiated contact. It has long been known that the amount of time a person spends with you can be an index of your significance to him. If he initiates and maintains eye contact, there is reason to believe that he is considering your requests and needs. If he pauses to chat or actually stops and talks, there is added reason to infer that he is individuating you. In four hospitals, the pseudopatient approached the staff member with a request which took the following form: "Pardon me, Mr. [or Dr. or Mrs.] X, could you tell me when I will be eligible for grounds privileges?" (or " . . . when I will be presented at the staff meeting?" or ". . . when I am likely to be discharged?"). While the content of the question varied according to the appropriateness of the target and the pseudopatient's (apparent) current needs the form was always a courteous and relevant request for information. Care was taken never to approach a particular member of the staff more than once a day, lest the staff member become suspicious or irritated. In examining these data, remember that the behavior of the pseudopatients was neither bizarre nor disruptive. One could indeed engage in good conversation with them.

The data for these experiments are shown in Table 1, separately for physicians (column 1) and for nurses and attendants (column 2). Minor differences between these four institutions were overwhelmed by the degree to which staff avoided continuing contacts that patients had initiated. By far, their most common response consisted of either a brief response to the question, offered while they were "on the move" and with head averted, or no response at all.

The encounter frequently took the following bizarre form: (pseudopatient) "Pardon me, Dr. X. Could you tell me when I am eligible for grounds privileges?" (physician) "Good morning, Dave. How are you today?" (Moves off without waiting for a response.)

It is instructive to compare these data with data recently obtained at Stanford University. It has been alleged that large and eminent universities are characterized by faculty who are so busy that they have no time for students. For this comparison, a young lady approached individual faculty members who seemed to be walking purposefully to some meeting or teaching engagement and asked them the following six questions.

1. "Pardon me, could you direct me to Encina Hall?" (at the medical school: ". . . to the Clinical Research Center?").
2. "Do you know where Fish Annex is?" (there is no Fish Annex at Stanford).
3. "Do you teach here?"
4. "How does one apply for admission to the college?" (at the medical school: ". . . to the medical school?").

TABLE 1. SELF-INITIATED CONTACT BY PSEUDOPATIENTS WITH PSYCHIATRISTS AND NURSES AND ATTENDANTS, COMPARED TO CONTACT WITH OTHER GROUPS.

Contact	*Psychiatric Hospitals*		*University Campus (Nonmedical)*	*University Medical Center*		
				Physicians		
	(1) Psychiatrists	*(2) Nurses and Attendants*	*(3) Faculty*	*(4) "Looking for a Psychiatrist"*	*(5) "Looking for an Internist"*	*(6) No Additional Comment*
Responses						
Moves on, head averted (%)	71	88	0	0	0	0
Makes eye contact (%)	23	10	0	11	0	0
Pauses and chats (%)	2	2	0	11	0	10
Stops and talks (%)	4	0.5	100	78	100	90
Mean number of questions answered (out of 6)	*	*	6	3.8	4.8	4.5
Respondents (No.)	13	47	14	18	15	10
Attempts (No.)	185	1283	14	18	15	10

*Not applicable.

5. "Is it difficult to get in?"
6. "Is there financial aid?"

Without exception, as can be seen in Table 1 (column 3), all of the questions were answered. No matter how rushed they were, all respondents not only maintained eye contact, but stopped to talk. Indeed, many of the respondents went out of their way to direct or take the questioner to the office she was seeking, to try to locate "Fish Annex," or to discuss with her the possibilities of being admitted to the university.

Similar data, also shown in Table 1 (columns 4, 5, and 6), were obtained in the hospital. Here too, the young lady came prepared with six questions. After the first question, however, she remarked to 18 of her respondents (column 4), "I'm looking for a psychiatrist," and to 15 others (column 5), "I'm looking for an internist." Ten other respondents received no inserted comment (column 6). The general degree of cooperative responses is considerably higher for these university groups than it was for pseudopatients in psychiatric hospitals. Even so, differences are apparent within the medical school setting. Once having indicated that she was looking for a psychiatrist, the degree of cooperation elicited was less than when she sought an internist.

POWERLESSNESS AND DEPERSONALIZATION

Eye contact and verbal contact reflect concern and individuation; their absence, avoidance and depersonalization. The data I have presented do not do justice to the rich daily encounters that grew up around matters of depersonalization and avoidance. I have records of patients who were beaten by staff for the sin of having initiated verbal contact. During my own experience, for example, one patient was beaten in the presence of other patients for having approached an attendant and told him, "I like you." Occasionally, punishment meted out to patients for misdemeanors seemed so excessive that it could not be justified by the most radical interpretations of psychiatric canon. Nevertheless, they appeared to go unquestioned. Tempers were often short. A patient who had not heard a call for medication would be roundly excoriated, and the morning attendants would often wake patients with. "Come on, you m-----f-----s, out of bed!"

Neither anecdotal nor "hard" data can convey the overwhelming sense of powerlessness which invades the individual as he is continually exposed to the depersonalization of the psychiatric hospital. It hardly matters *which* psychiatric hospital—the excellent public ones and the very plush private hospital were better than the rural and shabby ones in this regard, but again, the features that psychiatric hospitals had in common overwhelmed by far their apparent differences.

Powerlessness was evident everywhere. The patient is deprived of many of his legal rights by dint of his psychiatric commitment (*21*). He is shorn of credibility by virtue of his psychiatric label. His freedom of movement is restricted. He cannot initiate contact with the staff, but may only respond to such overtures as they make. Personal privacy is minimal. Patient quarters and possessions can be entered and examined by any staff member, for whatever reason. His personal history and anguish is available to any staff member (often including the "grey lady" and "candy striper" volunteer) who chooses to read his folder, regardless of their therapeutic relationship to him. His personal hygiene and waste evacuation are often monitored. The water closets may have no doors.

At times, depersonalization reached such proportions that pseudopatients had the sense that they were invisible, or at least unworthy of account. Upon being admitted, I and other pseudopatients took the initial physical examinations in a semipublic room, where staff members went about their own business as if we were not there.

On the ward, attendants delivered verbal and occasionally serious physical abuse to patients in the presence of other observing patients, some of whom (the pseudopatients) were writing it all down. Abusive behavior, on the other hand, terminated quite abruptly when other staff members were known to be coming. Staff are credible witnesses. Patients are not.

A nurse unbuttoned her uniform to adjust her brassiere in the presence of an entire ward of viewing men. One did not have the sense that she was being seductive. Rather, she didn't notice us. A group of staff persons might point to a patient in the dayroom and discuss him animatedly, as if he were not there.

One illuminating instance of depersonalization and invisibility occurred with regard to medications. All told, the pseudopatients were administered nearly 2100 pills, including Elavil, Stelazine, Compazine, and Thorazine, to name but a few. (That such a variety of medications should have been administered to patients presenting identical symptoms is itself worthy of note.) Only two were swallowed. The rest were either pocketed or deposited in the toilet. The pseudopatients were not alone in this. Although I have no precise records on how many patients rejected their medications, the pseudopatients frequently found the medications of other patients in the toilet before they deposited their own. As long as they were cooperative, their behavior and the pseudopatients' own in this matter, as in other important matters, went unnoticed throughout.

Reactions to such depersonalization among pseudopatients were intense. Although they had come to the hospital as participant ob-observers and were fully aware that they did not "belong," they nevertheless found themselves caught up in and fighting the process of depersonalization. Some examples: a graduate student in psychology asked his wife to bring his textbooks to the hospital so he could "catch up on his homework"—this despite the elaborate precautions taken to conceal his professional association. The same student, who had trained for quite some time to get into the hospital, and who had looked forward to the experience, "remembered" some drag races that he had wanted to see on the weekend and insisted that he be discharged by that time. Another pseudopatient attempted a romance with a nurse. Subsequently, he informed the staff that he was applying for admission to graduate school in psychology and was very likely to be admitted, since a graduate professor was one of his regular hospital visitors. The same person began to engage in psychotherapy with other patients—all of this as a way of becoming a person in an impersonal environment.

THE SOURCES OF DEPERSONALIZATION

What are the origins of depersonalization? I have already mentioned two. First are attitudes held by all of us toward the mentally ill—including those who treat them—attitudes characterized by fear, distrust, and horrible expectations on the one hand, and benevolent intentions on the other. Our ambivalence leads, in this instance as in others, to avoidance.

Second, and not entirely separate, the hierarchical structure of the psychiatric hospital facilitates depersonalization. Those who are at the top have least to do with patients, and their behavior inspires the rest of the staff. Average daily contact with psychiatrists, psychologists, residents, and physicians combined ranged from 3.9 to 25.1 minutes, with an overall mean of 6.8 (six pseudopatients over a total of 129 days of hospitalization). Included in this average are time spent in the admissions interview, ward meetings in the presence of a senior staff member, group and individual psychotherapy contacts, case presentation conferences, and discharge meetings. Clearly, patients do not spend much time in interpersonal contact with doctoral staff. And doctoral staff serve as models for nurses and attendants.

There are probably other sources. Psychiatric installations are presently in serious financial straits. Staff shortages are pervasive, staff time at a premium. Something has to give, and that something is patient contact. Yet, while financial stresses are realities, too much can be made of them. I have the impression that the psychological forces that result in depersonalization are much stronger than the fiscal ones and that the addition of more staff would not correspondingly improve patient care in this regard. The incidence of staff meetings and the enormous amount of record-keeping on patients, for example, have not been as substantially reduced as has patient contact. Priorities exist, even during hard times. Patient contact is not a significant priority in the traditional psychiatric hospital, and fiscal pressures do not account for this. Avoidance and depersonalization may.

Heavy reliance upon psychotropic medication tacitly contributes to depersonalization by convincing staff that treatment is indeed being conducted and that further patient contact may not be necessary. Even here, however, caution needs to be exercised in understanding the role of psychotropic drugs. If patients were powerful rather than powerless, if they were viewed as interesting individuals rather than diagnostic entities, if they were socially significant rather than social lepers, if their anguish truly and wholly compelled our sympathies and concerns, would we not *seek* contact with them, despite the availability of medications? Perhaps for the pleasure of it all?

THE CONSEQUENCES OF LABELING AND DEPERSONALIZATION

Whenever the ratio of what is known to what needs to be known approaches zero, we tend to invent "knowledge" and assume that we understand more than we actually do. We seem unable to acknowledge that we simply don't know. The needs for diagnosis and remediation of behavioral and emotional problems are enormous. But rather than acknowledge that we are just embarking on understanding, we continue to label patients "schizophrenic," "manic-depressive," and "insane," as if in those words we had captured the essence of understanding. The facts of the matter are that we have known for a long time that diagnoses are often not useful or reliable, but we have nevertheless continued to use them. We now know that we cannot distinguish insanity from sanity. It is depressing to consider how that information will be used.

Not merely depressing, but frightening. How many people, one wonders, are sane but not recognized as such in our psychiatric institutions? How many have been needlessly stripped of their privileges of citizenship, from the right to vote and drive to that of handling their own accounts? How many have feigned insanity in order to avoid the criminal consequences of their behavior, and, conversely, how many would rather stand trial than live interminably in a psychiatric hospital—but are wrongly thought to be mentally ill? How many have been stigmatized by well-intentioned, but nevertheless erroneous, diagnoses? On the last point, recall again that a "type 2 error" in psychiatric diagnosis does not have the same consequences it does in medical diagnosis. A diagnosis of cancer that has been found to be in error is cause for celebration. But psychiatric diagnoses are rarely found to be in error. The label sticks, a mark of inadequacy forever.

Finally, how many patients might be "sane" outside the psychiatric hospital but seem insane in it—not because craziness resides in them, as it were, but because they are responding to a bizarre setting, one that may be unique to institutions which harbor nether people? Goffman (*4*) calls the process of socialization to such institutions "mortification"—an apt metaphor that includes the processes of depersonalization that have been described here. And while it is impossible to know whether the pseudopatients' responses to these processes are characteristic of all inmates—they were, after all, not real patients—it is difficult to believe that these processes of socialization to a psychiatric hospital provide useful attitudes or habits of response for living in the "real world."

SUMMARY AND CONCLUSIONS

It is clear that we cannot distinguish the sane from the insane in psychiatric hospitals. The hospital itself imposes a special environment in which the meanings of behavior can easily be misunderstood. The consequences to patients hospitalized in such an environment—the powerlessness, depersonalization, segregation, mortification, and self-labeling—seem undoubtedly countertherapeutic.

I do not, even now, understand this problem well enough to perceive solutions. But two matters seem to have some promise. The first concerns the proliferation of community mental health facilities, of crisis intervention centers, of the human potential movement, and of behavior therapies that, for all of their own problems, tend to avoid psychiatric labels, to focus on specific problems and behaviors, and to retain the individual in a relatively nonpejorative environment. Clearly, to the extent that we refrain from sending the distressed to insane places, our impressions of them are less likely to be distorted. (The risk of distorted perceptions, it seems to me, is always present, since we are much more sensitive to an individual's behaviors and verbalizations than we are to the subtle contextual stimuli that often promote them. At issue here is a matter of magnitude. And, as I have shown, the magnitude of distortion is exceedingly high in the extreme context that is a psychiatric hospital.)

The second matter that might prove promising speaks to the need to increase the sensitivity of mental health workers and researchers to the *Catch 22* position of psychiatric patients. Simply reading materials in this area will be of help to some such workers and researchers. For others, directly experiencing the impact of psychiatric hospitalization will be of enormous use. Clearly, further research into the social psychology of such total institutions will both facilitate treatment and deepen understanding.

I and the other pseudopatients in the psychiatric setting had distinctly negative reactions. We do not pretend to describe the subjective experiences of true patients. Theirs may be different from ours, particularly with the passage of time and the necessary process of adaptation to one's environment. But we can and do speak to the relatively more objective indices of treatment within the hospital. It could be a mistake, and a very unfortunate one, to consider that what happened to us derived from malice or stupidity on the part of the staff. Quite the contrary, our overwhelming impression of them was of people who really cared, who were committed and who were uncommonly intelligent. Where they failed, as they sometimes did painfully, it would be more accurate to attribute those failures to the environment in which they, too, found themselves than to personal callousness. Their perceptions and behavior were controlled by the situation rather than being motivated by a malicious disposition. In a more benign environment, one that was less attached to global diagnosis, their behaviors and judgments might have been more benign and effective.

REFERENCES AND NOTES

1. P. Ash, *J. Abnorm. Soc. Psychol.* 44, 272 (1949); A. T. Beck, *Amer. J. Psychiat.* 119, 210 (1962); A. T. Boisen, *Psychiatry* 2, 233 (1938); N. Kreitman, *J. Ment. Sci.* 107, 876 (1961); N. Kreitman, P. Sainsbury, J. Morrisey, J. Towers, J. Scrivener, *ibid.*, p. 887; H. O. Schmitt and C. P. Fonda, *J. Abnorm. Soc. Psychol.* 52, 262 (1956); W. Seeman, *J. Nerv. Ment. Dis.* 118, 541 (1953). For an analysis of these artifacts and summaries of the disputes, see J. Zubin, *Annu. Rev. Psychol.* 18, 373 (1967); L. Phillips and J. G. Draguns, *ibid.* 22, 447 (1971).
2. R. Benedict, *J. Gen. Psychol.* 10, 59 (1934).
3. See in this regard H. Becker, *Outsiders: Studies in the Sociology of Deviance* (Free Press, New York, 1963); B. M. Braginsky,

D. D. Braginsky, K. Ring, *Methods of Madness: The Mental Hospital as a Last Resort* (Holt, Rinehart & Winston, New York, 1969); G. M. Crocetti and P. V. Lemkau, *Amer. Sociol. Rev.* 30, 577 (1965); E. Goffman, *Behavior in Public Places* (Free Press, New York, 1964); R. D. Laing, *The Divided Self: A Study of Sanity and Madness* (Quadrangle, Chicago, 1960); D. L. Phillips, *Amer. Sociol. Rev.* 28, 963 (1963); T. R. Sarbin, *Psychol. Today* 6, 18 (1972); E. Schur, *Amer. J. Sociol.* 75, 309 (1969); T. Szasz, *Law, Liberty and Psychiatry* (Macmillan, New York, 1963); *The Myth of Mental Illness: Foundations of a Theory of Mental Illness* (Hoeber-Harper, New York, 1963). For a critque of some of these views, see W. R. Grove, *Amer. Sociol. Rev.* 35, 873 (1970).

4. E. Goffman, *Asylums* (Doubleday, Garden City, N.Y., 1961).
5. T. J. Scheff, *Being Mentally Ill: A Sociological Theory* (Aldine, Chicago, 1966).
6. Data from a ninth pseudopatient are not incorporated in this report because, although his sanity went undetected, he falsified aspects of his personal history, including his marital status and parental relationships. His experimental behaviors therefore were not identical to those of the other pseudopatients.
7. A. Barry, *Bellevue Is a State of Mind* (Harcourt Brace Jovanovich, New York, 1971); I. Belknap, *Human Problems of a State Mental Hospital* (McGraw-Hill, New York, 1956); W. Caudill, F. C. Redlich, H. R. Gilmore, E. B. Brody, *Amer. J. Orthopsychiat.* 22, 314 (1952); A. R. Goldman, R. H. Bohr, T. A. Steinberg, *Prof. Psychol.* 1, 427 (1970); unauthored, *Roche Report* 1 (No. 13), 8 (1971).
8. Beyond the personal difficulties that the pseudopatient is likely to experience in the hospital, there are legal and social ones that, combined, require considerable attention before entry. For example, once admitted to a psychiatric institution, it is difficult, if not impossible, to be discharged on short notice, state law to the contrary notwithstanding. I was not sensitive to these difficulties at the outset of the project, nor to the personal and situational emergencies that can arise, but later a writ of habeas corpus was prepared for each of the entering pseudopatients and an attorney was kept "on call" during every hospitalization. I am grateful to John Kaplan and Robert Bartels for legal advice and assistance in these matters.
9. However distasteful such concealment is, it was a necessary first step to examining these questions. Without concealment, there would have been no way to know how valid these experiences were; nor was there any way of knowing whether whatever detections occurred were a tribute to the diagnostic acumen of

the staff or to the hospital's rumor network. Obviously, since my concerns are general ones that cut across individual hospitals and staffs, I have respected their anonymity and have eliminated clues that might lead to their identification.

10. Interestingly, of the 12 admissions, 11 were diagnosed as schizophrenic and one, with the identical symptomatology, as manic-depressive psychosis. This diagnosis has a more favorable prognosis, and it was given by the only private hospital in our sample. On the relations between social class and psychiatric diagnosis, see A. deB. Hollingshead and F. C. Redlich, *Social Class and Mental Illness: A Community Study* (Wiley, New York, 1958).
11. It is possible, of course, that patients have quite broad latitudes in diagnosis and therefore are inclined to call many people sane, even those whose behavior is patently aberrant. However, although we have no hard data on this matter, it was our distinct impression that this was not the case. In many instances, patients not only singled us out for attention, but came to imitate our behaviors and styles.
12. J. Cumming and E. Cumming, *Community Ment. Health* 1, 135 (1965); A. Farina and K. Ring, *J. Abnorm. Psychol.* 70, 47 (1965); H. E. Freeman and O. G. Simmons, *The Mental Patient Comes Home* (Wiley, New York, 1963); W. J. Johannsen, *Ment. Hygiene* 53, 218 (1969); A. S. Linsky, *Soc. Psychiat.* 5, 166 (1970).
13. S. E. Asch, *J. Abnorm. Soc. Psychol.* 41, 258 (1946); *Social Psychology* (Prentice-Hall, New York, 1952).
14. See also I. N. Mensh and J. Wishner, *J. Personality* 16, 188 (1947); J. Wishner, *Psychol. Rev.* 67, 96 (1960); J. S. Bruner and R. Tagiuri, in *Handbook of Social Psychology*, G. Lindzey, Ed. (Addison-Wesley, Cambridge, Mass., 1954), vol. 2, pp. 634-654; J. S. Bruner, D. Shapiro, R. Tagiuri, in *Person Perception and Interpersonal Behavior*, R. Tagiuri and L. Petrullo, Eds. (Stanford Univ. Press, Stanford, Calif., 1958), pp. 277-288.
15. For an example of a similar self-fulfilling prophecy, in this instance dealing with the "central" trait of intelligence, see R. Rosenthal and L. Jacobson, *Pygmalion in the Classroom* (Holt, Rinehart & Winston, New York, 1968).
16. E. Zigler and L. Phillips, *J. Abnorm. Soc. Psychol.* 63, 69 (1961). See also R. K. Freudenberg and J. P. Robertson, *A.M.A. Arch. Neurol. Psychiatr.* 76, 14 (1956).
17. W. Mischel, *Personality and Assessment* (Wiley, New York, 1968).
18. The most recent and unfortunate instance of this tenet is that of Senator Thomas Eagleton.

19. T. R. Sarbin and J. C. Mancuso, *J. Clin. Consult. Psychol.* 35, 159 (1970); T. R. Sarbin, *ibid.* 31, 447 (1967); J. C. Nunnally, Jr., *Popular Conceptions of Mental Health* (Holt, Rinehart & Winston, New York, 1961).
20. A. H. Stanton and M. S. Schwartz, *The Mental Hospital: A Study of Institutional Participation in Psychiatric Illness and Treatment* (Basic, New York, 1954).
21. D. B. Wexler and S. E. Scoville, *Ariz. Law Rev.* 13, 1 (1971).
22. I thank W. Mischel, E. Orne, and M. S. Rosenhan for comments on an earlier draft of this manuscript.

Delivery Patterns and Reproductive Efficiency in Groups of Negro and Caucasian Women

MARY JO KASSLEMAN

The following brief report is in distinct contrast to the previous articles in this section. Kasselman views transcultural nursing from the frame of reference of comparative anatomy. Are there differences in labor and delivery patterns across ethnic lines? If class is held constant, is there any difference between Caucasian Americans and Black Americans? Her data-collection method could be duplicated for other ethnic minorities. This paper exemplifies the uses to which the theories and methods of physical anthropology can be put. Also, the clarity of the research controls and the clear-cut measurable criteria differ from the more subjective data obtained by participant-observation.

For those who are interested in population studies no issue is of more vital concern than the future number of live births. The concern of health workers regarding this issue stems from the wish to insure the survival of dwindling populations and to provide adequate health care for future generations. It is thus important that we be able to predict future pregnancy outcomes with accuracy.

An original paper. By permission of the author.

In the United States it is accepted that there are measurable differences between newborn nonwhite and newborn white infants. For example, the average size of Negro infants is smaller at term than the Caucasian; there is also a higher incidence of prematurity and perinatal mortality in the former group. There is substantial evidence that the differences arise from a combination of biological and socioeconomic factors. Confusion in explaining or understanding these differences arises only when one looks for evidence that the observed differences are primarily racial in nature or that the differences represent instead principally socioeconomic phenomena.

Numerous studies have indicated that the observed differences are socioeconomic in origin. There is also evidence to suggest that some differences are racial in association. Seemingly conflicting findings from study to study have resulted in varied methodologies. Sample-selection procedures and criteria used to evaluate the progress and outcomes of pregnancy for the mother and the infant vary with the investigator.

Problem: The study was designed to demonstrate differences in delivery patterns and reproductive efficiency that are identifiable as of probable racial association, between a group of Negro and a group of Caucasian mothers and their infants.

Significance of the Problem: The epidemiological approach used for this study should contribute to elucidating the sources and mechanisms of any differences in delivery patterns and reproductive efficiency. Steps can be taken (e.g., early diagnosis, improved prognosis with proper therapy), to modify the expression of race-associated tendencies if it is possible to identify potentially high-risk populations. Therefore, knowledge of host or personal characteristics in disease can greatly benefit an individual or group.

Sample: The sample was selected from patients admitted to the Department of Obstetrics and Gynecology Outpatient Clinic at the Kansas University Medical Center in Kansas City, Kansas. To demonstrate any racial differences that might exist it was important to control, as much as possible, socioeconomic and medically complicating factors. Thus, the 139 Caucasian and 127 Negro women in the sample were selected and controlled for the following factors: 1) established pregnancy with the expectation of delivery in the calendar year 1970, 2) age between 18 and 30 for the 1970 pregnancy, 3) marital status—married for the 1970 pregnancy, and 4) 1970 socioeconomic status—both groups were classified as lower middle class on the Hollingshead Two-Factor Index of Social Position.

Methodology: Data were collected, from clinical records and interviews, on the women and all of their infants and pregnancies up to and including the 1970 pregnancy so that some within-group comparisons to the 1970 pregnancy could be made. Data on the following variables were collected: 1) birth order of each woman's pregnancy, 2) mother's Ponderal Index, the height divided by the cube root of the weight, for the 1970 pregnancy, 3) age of the mothers at each of their pregnancies, 4) trimester of each pregnancy that each woman began receiving medical care, 5) trimester of each pregnancy when ante-partal death of the fetus occurred, 6) ante-partal maternal complications for each pregnancy, 7) length of labor for each pregnancy, 8) occurrence of immediate post-partum maternal complications, 9) sex of each infant, 10) weight of each infant, 11) total length of each infant, 12) crown rump length of each infant, 13) biparietal width of each infant's head, 14) head circumference of each infant, 15) chest circumference of each infant, 16) Apgar scores at five minutes after birth of each infant, and 17) each infant's condition in the early neonatal period.

Data Analysis: Data collected describing the sample were analyzed using the following approaches: 1) Means, ranges, standard deviations, and standard error of the means were computed for all the variables of the women in the total sample and all their pregnancies. Means, etc., were also computed for both racial groups in the total sample. 2) Correlation coefficients were determined between all the variables for the total sample of women and pregnancies and for both racial groups in the total sample. 3) Frequency distributions of all variables for both racial groups of the total sample were obtained. 4) An F test was used to determine whether significant differences existed between the means of the variable in both groups in the total sample. 5) Means, ranges, standard deviations, and standard error of the means were computed for all the variables for all the mothers (using the five control factors) and their 1970 infants. 6) Frequency distributions of the variables for both racial groups in the 1970 sample were obtained. 7) A Chi square test was used to determine whether the frequency of all the variables differed significantly between racial groups in the 1970 portion of the sample.

Findings and Implications: The differences in the variables of the total sample where the five control factors were not used, were expected and did appear. Such things as significant differences in maternal age, infant weight, length, head and chest circumference, Apgar scores, and condition post-partum appeared. The Negro mothers were younger for their pregnancies and their infants smaller. However, in the controlled 1970 sample the only difference of significance was in the weight of the infants. The Negro infant weight mean was 217 grams less than the Caucasian infant weight mean.

The data analysis supports the assertion that if the factors used for controls in this study are employed, pregnancy outcomes in Negro and Caucasian women will differ only by weight of the infants. The slightly lower weight of the black infant at birth does not seem to represent lessened vigor. The implications of this study for health workers engaged in the care and counseling of pregnant women are clear.

Further study employing gross genetic controls of the sample seem indicated. Also, more information about nutritional patterns in the sample might shed further light on the reason for the weight differences in the infants.

COMPARATIVE FINDING FOR GROUPS OF NEGRO AND CAUCASIAN WOMEN

Caucasians	*Negroes*
1. The infant born in 1970 is this woman's second child.	1. Same.
2. The parents' index of social position is on the lower middle socioeconomic level.	2. Same.
3. Her ponderal index is 12.5 indicating a height of 5 feet and 5 to 6 inches and weight of 120 to 130 pounds.	3. Same.
4. Her age at the 1970 delivery was 22.8 years.	4. Her age at the 1970 delivery was 22.0 years.
5. She was more likely to seek medical care for the 1970 pregnancy in the latter part of the first trimester. 0.1 significance.*	5. She was more likely to seek medical care for the 1970 pregnancy in the early part of the second trimester.
6. She had a high probability of completing this 1970 pregnancy successfully.	6. Same.
7. If maternal complications antepartum were present they tended to be of mild nature.	7. Same.
8. The mean length of labor was 9 hours.	8. Mean length of labor was 9.2 hours (variability greater but no significant difference).
9. She was unlikely to have severe maternal post-partum complications but may have more mild complications. 0.05 significance.*	9. Unlikely to have maternal post-partum complications.
10. She had a very slightly larger probability of having a male infant in this 1970 pregnancy. 0.1 significance.*	10. She had a very slightly larger probability of having a female infant in this 1970 pregnancy.
11. The weight of the infant was 3370 grams or 7 pounds 3 ounces. 0.01 significance.*	11. The weight of the infant was 3153 grams or 6 pounds and 11 ounces.
12. The total length of the infant was 51 centimeters or 20 inches.	12. The total length of the infant was 49.9 centimeters or 19.9 inches.
13. Crown rump length was 32.1 centimeters or 12.5 inches.	13. Same.
14. Biparietal width was 9.9 centimeters or 3.9 inches. 0.01 significance.*	14. Biparietal width was 9.7 centimeters or 3.8 inches. (A number of infants in this group had biparietal measurements in the smaller ranges.)

Caucasians	*Negroes*
15. The head circumference was 34.6 centimeters or 13.8 inches.	15. 34.1 centimeters.
16. The chest circumference was 33.7 centimeters or 13.4 inches.	16. 33.5 centimeters.
17. Apgar score was 9.6 representing virtually no infant impairment at birth.	17. Same.
18. The infant's condition post-partum represents an uneventful early neonatal period.	18. Same.

*Significant difference

Unleashing the Untrained: Some Observations on Student Ethnographers

JAMES E. MYERS

Myers describes the pitfalls that await the beginner in participant-observation. Just as in any other method of data collection, and perhaps more so, the novice must be aware of his possible infringement of human rights—particularly the right to privacy. Is the research goal to satisfy the curiosity of the researcher? Are the methods and strategies appropriate to the purpose of the study? Although the papers discussed by Myers were written by anthropology students, the topics and data-collection methods are similar to those found in clinical papers written by nursing students.

Myers' article also illustrates the range of topics that could be studied by nursing students. For example, nurses could study segments of the population that have differing health needs: communes, nudist camps, retirement communities, migrant camps, skid rows, and so on. Or nurses could study the transexual patient, the heroin addict, or the suicide. Groups such as Hare Krishna, Gypsies, reservation Indians, or Christian Scientists also could be examined for their health care needs. All segments of the population are potential, if not actual, patients. Their needs, their beliefs, and their health behavior may differ from that of the nurse and may require a different approach to the nursing process. The uses to which participant-

Reproduced by permission of the Society for Applied Anthropology from ***Human Organization*** 28, No. 2 (1969):155-59.

observation can be put are as great as there are different cultural and subcultural groups with which the nurse can interact.

Like many other colleges and universities in the United States, Chico State College in California offers an upper-division anthropology course in "Comparative Societies." As elsewhere, the course description in the College catalog is sufficiently general and ambiguous to allow a broad interpretation of what constitutes appropriate content. Most importantly for this paper, it affords the instructor considerable freedom in determining what sort of term project he wants to try to pry loose from sometimes reluctant students.

During the first week of class in the fall of 1967, and before I had made any firm decision to require what probably would have been a typical library research paper, a lively class discussion developed around the subject of gathering anthropological field data. Encouraged by what struck me as a rather cavalier attitude on the part of the more vocal members of the class toward the enthnographer's task of gathering data in his own as well as other cultures, I assigned each student the semester-long task of gathering field data on a subject of his own choice.

For practical reasons, the assignment did not follow the broad *Notes and Queries on Anthropology* format.[1] The limitations of time required that the students select, observe, and analyze a specific behavior, event, or institution on the campus or in the community. The primary goal was to give them an opportunity to experience on a microscale some of the problems confronting the anthropologist seeking information from human beings about human beings. The methodological emphasis was on the nose-to-nose confrontation inherent in various participant-observation situations, and the students were informed that papers would be evaluated primarily in terms of evidence showing their achievement of skills directly related to various participant-observer problems. Thus, entrée into the field, structuring of the observer's role, and sequence and timing of observation took precedence over definitions of problems, generation and validation of hypotheses, control of variables, and other traditional aspects of scientific problem solving.

For three class meetings I presented lecture material to illustrate the notion that people often are not able to tell a researcher why or what they are doing or believe, either because they do not know, or (and more beguiling) because they consciously or unconsciously distort facts, withhold data, or otherwise confound the ethnographer. The students were reminded that the difference between stated belief and observed behavior may be especially difficult to sort out when the information being sought lies in an area culturally regarded as "controversial" or "sensitive." During this time I relied heavily on material from my own field experiences and from two excellent articles on field work problems by Paul and by Becker and Geer.[2]

Before describing the types of problems tackled by these intrepid ethnographers, several general points should be made:

1. During the first semester the assignment was given, there were no anthropology majors in the class of 50 students—simply because there was no B.A. program in anthropology at the time. During the second semester, after anthropology had become a bachelor's program, five anthropology majors were enrolled in the class of 48 students. These five were majors only by the fact of declaration and actually possessed a very meager background in anthropology.
2. Except for the three introductory lectures on selected field work problems, no further instruction on the problems and techniques of gathering data in the field was provided, and the students were essentially on their own.
3. It would undoubtedly appear more professional if I could report that my laissez-faire approach to the assignment was governed by a cleverly conceived pedagogical hypothesis designed to instill in students the value of independent research. The fact is, although initially harboring every intention of providing supervision for the students, I was so swamped with other academic and administrative work for the two semesters the course was given that the effect was to unleash on the college community 98 curious and enthusiastic, but notably untrained and unsupervised student ethnographers.

CATEGORIES OF RESEARCH SELECTED

Ninety-one of the original 98 students completed the task. Of the seven who did not, three failed even to venture into the field, two gathered their data but were unable to produce a manuscript, one gathered data but claimed to have lost his "extensive" field notes to a thief, and one student failed to return from his field excursion to the Haight-Ashbury.

The problems studied fell into eight major categories:

1. *Womb-to-Tomb Critical Events.* This was the single largest category, with 21 students observing the most important

ceremonies, events, and ritual behaviors occuring in an individual's life cycle (birthdays, betrothals, weddings, divorces, and funerals).

2. *The Religious World.* Seventeen students trained their energies on various religious ceremonies and beliefs (Roman Catholic mass, Jehovah Witnesses, St. Germaine Society, the priesthood, the Holy Eucharist).
3. *The Body Beautiful.* Fourteen field workers explored the mysteries surrounding the care and nurturing of the human body and the various types of attention it receives by the owner and by the spectator. (Female figure, beauty parlor, ear piercing, sorority girls and their breasts.)
4. *Fun and Games.* Thirteen people sought to understand the behavior associated with organized recreation. Reflecting their own career interests to a degree greater than any other category, all thirteen were from the Physical Education Department. (Football, surfing, golfing, automobile racing, the keg party.)
5. *The World of Work.* Nine students ventured into occupational areas, seeking to understand how and why man earns his bread and keep. (The car salesman, the life insurance salesman, the Negro hustler, the mailman.)
6. *Associations.* College fraternities and sororities, community clubs, and other nonkinship sodalities were studied by six students. (John Birch Society, the Boy Scouts, behavioral norms at a fraternity house, the Free Masons, the pledge role in the Lambda Pi fraternity.)
7. *Social Problems.* Seven papers were directed toward social problems in the community and on the campus. (The drunk, the collegiate user of marijuana, homosexuals, three juvenile delinquents, abortion.)
8. *Miscellanea.* This catch-all category comprised numerous research topics too varied to assign to any of the other areas. (Contraceptive buying, a Negro speech community, toilet behavior of the college student, seating arrangements in the College Union.)

Twenty-three students (25 percent of the class) directed their research to on-campus situations. Nine students (10 percent of the class) plunged into research areas that would be designated as culturally sensitive, i.e., they purposely selected topics demanding the utmost in observational and/or interviewing skills—for example, the papers on contraceptive purchasing, homosexuality, breasts, hustling, abortion, unmarried couples living together, pot and drugs on campus.

Fifty-nine students (54 percent) approached their problem by declaring their role of observer, 34 students (38 percent) were already members of the group they selected to study, and eight students (9 percent) decided it advantageous to pose as a member of the group being studied, although in fact they were not.

SOME SAMPLE FINDINGS

In addition to the wide variety of research subjects chosen, the students displayed immense variation in the style, approach, and quality of their papers. The following brief excerpts and descriptions represent neither the best nor the poorest papers, nor do they represent the most seriously motivated students. They have been selected merely to convey the creativity that can be obtained from students unfettered by the restricting bonds of training and supervision.

In a paper entitled "The Keg Party," one student studied a peculiar type of campus corroboree known as the "kegger," or keg party. Based on his attendance at thirteen keggers held during one semester, the participant-observer clearly spent more time participating than observing. However, the descriptive quality of his paper was good, and the reader emerges with a feeling that an Erik Erikson has done some reinterpreting of Allan Holmberg's happy description of a Siriono drinking bout:

> The keg is usually carried to the party site by the persons who purchased it, and there seems to be some status involved in triumphantly bringing this prize into the party area. There is an immediate uproar with the arrival of the keg, and people quickly go to work preparing for the festivities. The keg itself is a large aluminum container of some thickness which stand 2.5 feet tall with a circumference of about three feet at its widest point. It is filled with a beverage called beer, which has an alcoholic content of approximately 4.5 percent. The tapping process is usually attended to by a person who is respected because of his experience and expert handling of the process. The tapper has command and authority over the party at this point and the people follow his directions in order to finish with the work and get the beer flowing. The keg location is clearly the center of the party. The keg itself is almost given the place of a totem, notice the widespread excitement as it is brought in and made ready for tapping. This observer wonders about the possibility of the tap being a phallic symbol; witness the plunging of the cylindrical shaft into the round, awaiting container, and the cheers that go up when the liquid spurts forth.

Incidentally, this student fondness for pop-psych as an analytical tool was evident in a half-dozen papers.

Without a doubt the acme of observational skills was reached in a paper entitled "Toilet Behavior of the College Student." Recognizing that all peoples enact certain rituals to maintain their aplomb during the act of voiding, and that American society confines urination and defecation to certain rooms and fixtures, the student proceeded to analyze the behavior of males and females using first and second floor toilets in one building on the campus. Showing the advantage of having the spouse accompany the anthropologist into the field, the student ethnographer, with the unflagging and devoted aid of his wife, became privy to data that resulted in this reporter's public bathroom performance being affected forever.

The paper contained excellent diagrams of the toilet rooms observed. It included a telling analysis of urinal and stall choice, with impressive frequency distribution tables to lend statistical support to the commonly observed fact that men and women do not randomly select a stall or a urinal, as the case may be. With the sure hand of a veteran experimentalist, variable behavior was forced on the subjects by the researcher himself occupying select stall or urinals and then observing the results.

The observer concluded that self-consciousness is the major contributor to male/female toilet behavior. This was evidenced in many instances, but especially by the frequent faint-of-heart females who used the technique of waiting until one person flushed the toilet, and then urinating or defecating while the noise from the adjoining toilet drowned out the sounds of one's own relief; or, quickly relieving one's self and exiting before the stranger could see who was in the adjoining stall.

The class award for questionable motivation and hanky-panky under the guise of science, went to a fraternity lad who wrote a paper entitled, "My Cup Runneth Over: A Study of Sorority Girls and Their Breasts." Happily for science, his enthusiastic but unrealistic initial research ideas gave way to reality. After dismissing an impressive corps of eager male volunteer assistants, abandoning certain interesting techniques that had little significance to his stated problem, and enlisting the aid of female volunteer assistants to administer his questionnaire and conduct interviews, he turned out a respectable piece of research on beauty and the breast.

One student studied the activities and beliefs of ten Negro hustlers in one California metropolitan area for three months. Few students would have been able to study this subject successfully, but in this case the researcher himself came from a lower-lower class background and was familiar with his topic from prior experience. Apparently having no trouble drawing what in such a study could be an important methodological line between participation and observation, he "moved in and out of the scene with [his] hustler informants." Much of this student's success derived from the endorsements given him by two high-status hustlers, and his paper evidenced excellent observational and reporting skills in describing the hustlers' dwellings and furnishings, food, dress, grooming, violence, competition, and, of course, their women.

METHODOLOGICAL AND ETHICAL VIOLENCE

Relentless in their quest for information, some of the students exhibited a blatant disregard for the rights of others and frankly startled me with the ease and willingness by which they disclosed certain data obviously not intended to go beyond the point of original reception. For example:

1. *Disclosure of Secret Rituals.* Much was written about heretofore secret rites and ceremonies of various fraternities and sororities, both collegiate and community. Some of the information was wrestled from its owners by devious means and in some cases was proffered to the researcher only with the understanding it would not be disclosed to anyone else.
2. *Violation of Anonymity and Privacy.* One of the few caveats stressed in class in reference to the research was the great importance to be attached to informant and institutional anonymity when requested. This admonition was freqently violated and typically in those cases where anonymity and privacy was most important.
3. *The "Homing" Questionnaire.* Another unfortunate technique was the clever design and use of the "homing" questionnaire, i.e., questionnaires that clearly indicated "do not use names," but which nevertheless were surreptitiously keyed to allow the researcher to identify who filled out a particular questionnaire. In some cases the student's reason for the subterfuge was unclear; in other cases, e.g., the study of the sorority girls' breast and brassiere beliefs, the motivation—though not condoned—can be appreciated.
4. *Disclosure of Illegal Practices.* Some reports focused on illegal practices and thus contained information that would, if made public, activate campus and/or civil authorities.

5. *Misrepresentation.* Puzzling was the practice of some students who for one reason or another misrepresented themselves. Often overlooking the fact that the role of student would suffice to gain entrée and gather information, they proceeded under the guise of various false statuses.
6. *The Amateur Professional.* Frightening was the ease with which two junior students assumed the status of experienced professional and administered and analyzed various projective and intelligence tests in their study of a culturally disadvantaged family. One wrote: "I attempted to give her the Goodenough projective test . . . Next I attempted administering Murray's T.A.T. test . . . At this time I tried to give the daughter the sentence-completion test I had devised, but I learned she was unable to read . . . Next I tried the Rorschach Inkblot test."

UNFORESEEN RAMIFICATIONS

At least two students learned rather dramatically that social research can proceed down unintended and unforeseen avenues. Although the two examples of unplanned developments given here are a long way from DuBois' remembrances of her five unfortuante Alorese informants who were publicly decapitated by the Japanese as a warning to other informants, they are important in giving credence to her belief that "there is no end to the intricate chain of responsibility and guilt that the pursuit of even the most arcane social research involves."[3]

One student, for example, innocently set out to explore coffee-break behavior in a local county office. The result was a minor human relations catastrophe that undoubtedly involved her inexperienced approach as much as the fortuity of events that existed independent of her behavior. Thus, the study was poorly timed since a taxpayers' association was currently probing costs of county government, and was especially interested in unauthorized leaves and extended coffee breaks. The student also failed to gain approval for the study from appropriate personnel. This distressed certain administrators, who, themselves, were later charged by the taxpayers' association with not knowing what was going on under their very noses. Finally, she exhibited naiveté of organizational behavior ("I can't understand why 900 employees arose in anger and indignation when only 30 were directly involved").

Before the student realized what a tempest had been stirred up, three newspapers in the country had picked up the story ("Mysterious Coffee Break Survey"), the county employees' association distributed a flier urging all employees to beware of an unauthorized survey that threatened their coffee break, and the taxpayers' association was demanding further investigation into what appeared to be a typical county employee boondoggle of time.

The tragedy of the aborted study was summed up by an office informant:

> It is too bad that you had to walk right into the middle of an already difficult situation. It is sadder because you had no idea of the trouble you would cause. Your intentions were perfectly innocent, but you sure screwed things up.

Another student gathered data on community service clubs in a small town north of Chico. He minced few words concerning the discrepancy between one club's stated *raison d'etre* and what he actually observed, concluding that there was more "bulling and boozing" in the organization than anything else. A few weeks after he completed the study, a friend asked him if he could read it. He did—the entire paper—to the assembled members of the club. The members did not seem to appreciate this type of anthropological research and in fact indicated their intention of sending a formal complaint to the student, his instructor, and the college administration

CONCLUDING REMARKS

On the credit side of the assignment, undergraduate students at least had an opportunity to acquire an inkling of the problems and advantages of field work as a method of gathering data. On the debit side, some of the students probably wrought irreparable damage to future students who may also wish to use the community and the campus as a human research laboratory.

On the whole, however, the assignment has reinforced my positive feelings toward the importance of having undergraduate anthropology students pursue basic field training on the campus or in the community. Whether the student is going on to graduate studies or not, we are remiss if we do not see that he has some first-hand experience with the discipline's primary technique of gathering data.

The optimum learning experience would be an undergraduate course in field methodology, perhaps along the lines described by Bennett,[4] plus supervised work in the field with a trained enthnographer. When either of these is not possible, as is most often the case in undergraduate programs today, an improved version of what has been described here may be the best solution. Improvements might take many forms, but minimally, in order to avoid the problems cited in this paper, it would demand more hours devoted to classroom training and closer surveillance of the proposed studies.

NOTES AND REFERENCES

1. Royal Anthropological Institute of Great Britain and Ireland, *Notes and Queries on Anthropology*, (sixth ed.), Routledge and Kegan Paul, London, 1951.
2. Benjamin D. Paul, "Interview Techniques and Field Relationships," in *Anthropology Today*, University of Chicago Press, Chicago, 1953, pp. 430-475; Howard Becker and Blanche Geer, "Participant-Observation: The Analysis of Qualitative Field Data," in Richard Adams and Jack Preiss (eds.), *Human Organization Research*, The Dorsey Press, Homewood, Ill, 1960, pp. 267-289.
3. Cora DuBois, *The People of Alor*, Harper and Brothers, New York, 1960, p. xiv.
4. John Bennett, "Individual Perspective in Field Work: An Experimental Training Course," in Richard Adams and Jack Preiss (eds.), *op. cit.*, pp. 267-289.

Integration through Application

The application of anthropological theories and methods to the theory, research, and practice of nursing is still in an embryonic stage. As the cadre of nurse-anthropologists increases, and as they publish their findings in nursing journals, the knowledge base of transcultural nursing will be extended. However, and this must be strongly emphasized, nurse-anthropologists do not have exclusive rights to the field of transcultural nursing. Every nurse who uses her nursing process to discover the cultural variable is practicing transcultural nursing. Nursing case studies which focus on the cultural aspects of nursing care are a valid approach to theory building. Many more case studies are needed. Clinical nurses have a wealth of data at their fingertips not available to either nurse researchers or to anthropologists. It is the clinical base of nursing, which only a nurse can provide, that makes transcultural nursing a field separate from anthropology.

The integration of anthropological knowledge and skills with nursing is accomplished through nursing practice, research, education, consultation, and administration. At one time, nursing schools focused on integrating mental health concepts into the curriculum; a similar focus could be applied to integrate cultural concepts. Nurse anthropologists could be hired by schools of nursing to perform this task. Or, transcultural nurse experts could be consultants to nursing service or nursing education organizations to provide guidelines for the integration of cultural concepts. In-service education programs, or staff development, could focus upon a nursing care plan that would include the cultural variable.

A beginning step in integration is the examination of nursing itself. What are our beliefs about nurisng, nursing's contribution to health care, and nursing's expectations of patient behavior? As nurses, what are our variations in value orientation? What value orientations do we expect from patients? What are our communication systems? Do we use words that have meaning for patients, or even other nurses? As nurses, do we create a communication system intelligible only to ourselves? Do we impose our beliefs about health and illness on our patients, or do we attempt to discover their views first? Do our attitudes toward patients differ depending upon the patient's diagnosis, his compliance with the treatment regimen, or his ability to get well?

The second step is the study of patients. What are the patient's attitudes and beliefs about life and death, health and illness, medical and nursing care? What is the patient's variation in value orientation. His communication system? What is the patient's past history with the health care delivery system? Has it affected his current progress? How has he been socialized into the patient role? Has he used other health care systems in the past, or is he using one concurrently? What does the patient think of his nursing care? Since nursing's primary focus has always been on the patient, the addition of anthropological theory to the study of patients will add to nursing's knowledge base, rather than distract the nurse from this prime focus.

A third step is directed to the health care delivery system itself. What, again, are the belief systems held by our Western form of health care delivery? What are the behavioral requirements of its members? Who is an in-group member, and who is considered as part of the out-group? What is nursing's place within this system? What is the position of the patient? Or, what, in fact, is the place of the health care delivery system within the structure of the entire social system? How does the Western system of health care interact with the other health systems? Since nurses and patients interact within the health care delivery system, the beliefs and requirements of the system affect the interaction, and need to be part of the analysis.

The above questions are only a few that need to be asked and answered by nursing. In general, this book has been concerned with the nurse working within her own cultural context but who may come into contact with patients or other health professionals from different cultures. However, the nurse who works in a foreign country must ask the same questions but from a different perspective. Here the nurse, not the patient, is the outsider; and she is immediately confronted with differences in nursing, in patients, and in the health care delivery system. The nurse, believing that the way she was taught is the "right way," realizes that she is apt to be critical of what she sees simply because it is different. This clarity of vision can be developed by the domestic nurse working in her own culture. For both the foreign and domestic nurse, the values, beliefs, and rules of the health care delivery system must be viewed within its cultural context.

The papers in this section are research studies or research proposals based upon a particular patient population. The articles were chosen for their content, are predominantly descriptive, and reflect the state of transcultural nursing today. For the most part the papers do not emphasize nursing interventions, but rather add to nursing knowledge about a population or a patient problem in a crosscultural context.

Williams' paper is singular in this collection for its immediate applicability to nursing practice. Williams studied differences between Anglo and Mexican-American women in their response to hysterectomy as a surgical procedure. Although her study revealed few differences, her focus on convalescence as a valid area of nursing research makes her paper relatively unusual. Convalescence is poorly documented in our literature, yet it is primarily the responsibility of nursing. The great need for more research in this area with different populations is obvious.

In contrast, Annie Wauneka speaks of her experiences in a rural Navajo community and the need for clearer explanations to a recipient population. Health teaching, to whatever patient group, is an integral part of nursing, and the advice by Wauneka can be generalized to other peoples.

As we move again to an urban area, Louie discusses the acculturation process of the Chinese-American and provides us with insight into the blend of traditional Chinese thinking and American health beliefs. The process of assimilation of other nationalities into the American system, particularly in health and illness situations, is very sparse in the literature. The processes of linking and meshing might be found not just in Chinese but also in Armenians, Egyptians, or Argentinians. These concepts are worth looking at and testing.

"Terminal Care at Home in Two Cultures" compares and contrasts two culture groups rather than describing just one. This type of study provides us with more data for generalizations. But the study of Gypsy culture, as a "one of a kind" study, is critical to our understanding this little-known people. Dissimilar as they may seem, these two articles both reveal the warmth that develops between the researcher and the research subjects.

The last two papers are research proposals that follow the method of applied anthropology as discussed by Foster. From the New York Puerto Rican to the Arizona Papago, we can see the amount of information the nurse needs to know about the people with whom she intends to work in order to propose a nursing intervention. Both Winn and Brosnan have worked with "their people" and remain interested in them. The proposals indicate the need for greater data in the field.

As transcultural nursing develops into its own area of specialty more studies will become available. Nursing is in the position of being able to provide consumer-oriented studies more easily than any other field and should assist in raising the consciousness of the other health professions.

RECOMMENDED READINGS

Baca, Josephine Elizabeth. "Some Health Beliefs of the Spanish Speaking." *American Journal of Nursing* 69, No. 10 (1969): 2172-76.

Berkowitz, Philip, and Nancy S. Berkowitz, "The Jewish Patient in the Hospital," *American Journal of Nursing.* 67 (1967):2335-37.

Campbell, Theresa, and Betty Chang, "Health Care of the Chinese in America," *Nursing Outlook* 21, No. 4 (1973):245-49.

Johnson, Carmen Acosta, "Nursing and Mexican American Folk Medicine," *Nursing Forum* 3, No. 2 (1964):102-12.

Leininger, Madeleine, "Nursing Care of the Patient from Another Culture," *Nursing Clinics of North America* 2 (1967):747-62.

Loughlin, Bernice W., "Pregnancy in the Navaho Culture," *Nursing Outlook* 13, No. 3 (1965):55-58.

Moses, Marian, "Viva La Causa," *American Journal of Nursing* 73, No. 5 (1973):842-48.

Paynich, Mary Louise, "Cultural Barriers to Nurse Communication," *American Journal of Nursing* 64, No. 2 (1964):87-90.

Press, Irwin, "The Urban Currandero," *American Anthropologist* 73, No. 3 (1971):741-56.

Saunders, Lyle, *Cultural Differences and Medical Care.* New York: Russell Sage Foundation, 1954.

Zborowski, Mark, *People in Pain.* San Francisco: Jossey-Bass, Inc., Publishers, 1969.

Ethnocultural Responses to Hysterectomy: Implications for Nursing

MARGARET AASTERUD WILLIAMS

Williams uses the term ethnocultural to refer to the study of comparative values and beliefs held by ethnic minorities in the United States. This paper is based on research into second-generation Anglo and Mexican-American women post-hysterectomy. The reader is urged to obtain the entire dissertation from which the paper was abstracted, for a more complete discussion of the literature and of the research design. The integration of anthropology and nursing is clearly reflected in the problem selected and in the immediate applicability of the finding. More than any other, this paper exemplifies transcultural nursing research.

To what extent does a person's ethnocultural background influence how he will perceive and react to an illness or to treatment? Some persons in the health professions will say, "A great deal," and cite numerous examples to illustrate how cultural factors have, in their experience, seemed to profoundly influence illness behavior. Others

An original paper. By permission of the author. The unpublished dissertation is available through inter-library loan from the University of California, Berkeley. See the list of references at the end of the article.

will say, "Not at all; what seems to be characteristic of the responses of certain groups is really a matter of level of knowledge about health and illness, socioeconomic status, and the like." Still others will say, "Well, I think cultural factors are important, but I don't know just how."

This last, more tentative response may well be the best expression of the present state of knowledge regarding the influence of cultural factors in determining what persons define as illness; when (or if) they seek treatment; how they respond emotionally, physically and behaviorally to the illness and treatment; how health professionals are regarded; how the ill or convalescing person is regarded by family members; and so forth. Cultural factors are exceedingly difficult to separate from social or psychological factors in these considerations, and in fact, the relative influence of each is often a matter of conjecture.

Because of the ambiguity of cultural influence, health professionals may fall into one of two dichotomous ways of thinking about the matter; one based on the dictum, "Treat all patients alike, regardless of race, color, creed, or nationality"; the other based on the dictum, "Treat the patient as a unique person." The first, in its most extreme form, would imply that no particular consideration be given to cultural difference; the second, in its most extreme form, would imply that persons of particular ethnic descent or subcultural groups will be "different than" and require different treatment from persons of other groups. The susceptibility of the former way of thinking to routinized care and of the latter way of thinking to the development of stereotyping is obvious, yet the process may be insidious and may be rationalized on the basis of one of the foregoing dicta.

Persons of Mexican descent may be peculiarly vulnerable to stereotyping with respect to health care because of the characteristics of the literature available on their health beliefs and practices. Most of the studies have dealt with Mexican-American persons living in isolated, rural areas of the Southwest or in relatively unacculturated, lower-class ethnic enclaves within cities. The literature consequently has tended to emphasize the prevalence of folk beliefs and folk medicine and the caution, if not actual distrust, employed in dealing with Anglo health practitioners and agencies. The persistence of such beliefs and practices among second, third, or later generations living in urban areas is relatively unknown.

THE STUDY

These considerations, in addition to a long-standing interest in the reaction of women to hysterectomy, were the basis for a comparative study of convalescence post-hysterectomy among Mexican-American and Anglo women (1). The major assumption was that if two ethno-cultural groups could be kept as similar as possible in social and medical characteristics (and if personality was assumed to be related to cultural background), then possible differences in the perception of and response to diagnosis and treatment might well be on the basis of cultural background. During convalescence, for example, it seemed reasonable to assume that culturally transmitted beliefs and attitudes about illness and treatment and culturally patterned family relationships could be influential in determining what the person perceived as stressful, how he coped with discomfort, what type of and how much activity was engaged in, what attentions were given by family members, how closely medical instructions were followed, and how long the convalescence lasted.

The study therefore examined the relationship of the length of convalescence to ethnicity and perceived stress (separately and combined); it also examined variation in types of perceived stress between the two ethnic groups, and dealt with aspects of convalescent role behavior that included time of resumption of usual social role responsibilities, reliance on lay help and advice, and how closely medical instructions were followed. Stress was defined as the physical, social, and emotional difficulties or discomforts that the person reported undergoing during the experience, and convalescence was defined as that period of time extending from hospital discharge until the time indicated by the person as being when she felt fully recovered.

Sixty-four women (32 Anglo and 32 Mexican-American) living in three urban areas of northern California were interviewed at home at an average of nineteen weeks post-hospital discharge following vaginal or abdominal hysterectomies for nonmalignant pathology within the preceding seven months. (Hysterectomies performed for mental health reasons were excluded.) All Anglo respondents were third generation (native-born of native-born parents) or more and of northern European descent; all Mexican-American women were second generation (native-born of foreign-born or mixed parentage) or more. The groups were similar in marital status, in the number of persons employed occupationally, and in the number of days hospitalized. They were also similar in the type of hysterectomy performed, with approximately equal numbers in each group having undergone vaginal (including those with associated repairs) or abdominal hysterectomy (including those with associated salpingo-oophorectomies). Neither group occupationally exceeded lower white collar status or had more than a high school education. All women were pre-menopausal or peri-menopausal, with the average age of the Mexican-

American women being 35.8 years, that of the Anglo women being 33.4 years. Twenty-seven of the Mexican-American women were Catholic as compared to nine Anglo women. Their surgical procedures had been carried out in one private and two non-private hospitals. (Thirteen Anglo and eight Mexican-American women had private physicians.)

RESULTS OF STUDY

Since a description of the methods of data collection and data analysis are available elsewhere (2), only the results of the study that are most relevant to nursing care will be discussed here. The results indicated that length of convalescence was related to stress, but not significantly in a statistical sense, and there was no relationship to ethnicity as such. Both groups ended their convalescence at a median of eight weeks. (This length of time or less was considered to be a short-to-average convalescence; nine weeks or more was considered a long convalescence.) Increased age (36 years or more) appeared to be the most important factor in a longer convalescent period for both groups.

Variations occurred, however, in the extent of stress perceived by the two groups during both the preconvalescent and convalescent periods. With respect to the preconvalescent period, major areas of response dealt with what had been heard about the effect of a hysterectomy, possible religious concerns about having the operation, and possible concerns about their husbands' reactions. In response to the question, "What had you heard from other women about the good or bad effects of a hysterectomy?", many "old wives' tales" and bits of misinformation were cited, with a change for the worse in sexual relationships being high on the Mexican-American women's list, and emotional changes being high on the Anglo women's list. Examples of some of the phrases used with respect to the former were: "Empty"; "Half a woman"; "Husband doesn't like the woman anymore"; "Just like a shell." Examples of phrases used with respect to emotional changes were: "Get so nervous you're like crazy"; "Depressed"; "Lose one's mind"; "Cry all the time"; "Get hysterical when see babies." Other responses dealt with physical complications such as: "Gain weight"; "Always sick afterward"; "Feel older"; "Go through the change of life." Only three persons in each group said they had heard only about good effects (e.g., one would feel much better afterward, or that sexual relationships would be better); the rest had heard about the bad effects only or a combination of good and bad effects. One young woman said:

> People had me scared to death before surgery. They said, "You'll be nervous and screaming at the kids." I remember some saying you could get a nervous breakdown. One person who'd had the operation said I'd gain weight; another said I'd lose weight. Both of them said it would make me nervous. No one said anything about good effects.

Many of the women, of course, related lay information about after-effects but went on to say that they did not believe the stories or did not think they would be affected. Concerns about their husbands' reactions, however, appeared to be related in many instances to the tales. Twelve Mexican-American and eight Anglo women said that they had concerns about this, although no Anglo woman said that she had put off her surgery for this reason, as did several Mexican-American women. One person reported that she had needed, or at least wanted, this operation for eight years, but that her husband's signature on the operative permit had been required at other hospitals and he would not sign. (The hospital at which she finally had the surgery did not require the husband's signature—it was optional.) One woman, who was first generation and therefore not included in the main sample, had gone through the entire surgery, hospitalization, and convalescence without her husband knowing that it was a hysterectomy that had been performed; she had told him it was a hernia operation.

Only four persons in each group said that they had some religious concern about having this type of surgery or that they had talked to a priest about it. Many of the Catholic women who indicated no concern added statements to the effect that, "I knew it was for my own health." In general, then, religious concern appeared minimal among the Mexican-American women, but the number of Catholic Anglo women was too small to make comparison.

During convalescence the Mexican-American women tended to report the presence of somewhat more stressful physical and emotional symptoms that did the Anglo women, but the differences were not remarkable. Fourteen symptoms were inquired about:

1. Weakness or tiredness
2. Pain or discomfort
3. Bleeding,
4. Vaginal discharge
5. Bladder difficulties
6. Appetite or weight changes
7. Hot flashes
8. Feelings of "emptiness"

9. Feelings of being "full," "stuffed," or "sewn up"
10. Crying or tearfulness
11. Difficulty in concentrating
12. Nervousness
13. Irritability
14. Feelings of being "fragile"

More than half the women in both groups stated that they experienced more feelings of nervousness during convalescence than they had before surgery, and that they had feelings of being "fragile"; that is, they were afraid of being bumped or jarred in some way. Half or more of the Mexican-American women, but less than half the Anglo women said that:

1. They had bladder difficulties at home, either from the presence of a catheter, a urinary infection, or feelings of urgency or frequency.
2. They had "quite a bit" or "a lot" of weakness or tiredness or were in bed at home for over a week (as opposed to "not much", or being up and around almost as soon as they were home).
3. They had hot flashes at one time or another during convalescence.
4. They had episodes of crying, tearfulness, or "blueness" during convalescence that were unusual for them compared to before surgery.
5. They had some trouble with eating after they were home or had lost weight or gained weight—neither of which event they had wanted to occur.

Less than half of each group (six Anglos and fourteen Mexican-Americans) said that they experienced "quite a bit" of pain or discomfort after they were home from the hospital or took pain pills for more than two weeks, as opposed to "not much" or having taken pain pills for less than two weeks.

Other reactions which were considered as evidence of convalescent stress included missing having menstrual periods (by far the majority emphatically did not); sexual relationships not being as satisfactory as before surgery; worrying that removing the uterus would affect other body functions; finding some instructions hard to carry out; and wanting to call the physician but refraining from doing so. Little difference was found between the groups in these areas. Considering the apparent concern that Mexican-American women held before surgery about possible changes in sexual relationships, it is noteworthy that only seven persons said that relationships were actually less satisfactory afterward—the same number of Anglo women who also reported this. Stated otherwise, three-quarters of each group reported that there actually was no change or a change for the better in sexual relationships.

Respondents were also asked what was most troublesome to them during convalescence. Of interest is the fact that having to come home with a retention catheter was the major problem for only three out of ten Anglo women who had to cope with this accoutrement, but was the major problem for all ten of the Mexican-American women who came home with one. Anglo women, more than Mexican-American, tended to cite specific physical problems such as "shakiness," "soreness," "hard to sit down," and both groups had approximately equal numbers who found the activity restrictions or emotional problems the most troublesome.

With respect to convalescent role behavior, there was some evidence of cultural patterning. Household activities were resumed at a median of six weeks by the Mexican-American women and at four weeks by the Anglo women. Although it might be logical to ascribe this difference to the "help available," i.e., the Mexican-American women having more potential help from the larger number of children in the family and more female relatives, this would not appear to be the case. Eight Anglo women said they had very little help in contrast to only two Mexican-American women who said this, but again, this did not account for the two weeks' total difference. All but two of the Mexican-American women named family members as their main source of assistance; nine Anglo women mentioned neighbors or friends. (Husbands were equally supportive in household assistance in both groups.) It appeared, then, that illness rallied support in both groups, but that it was more often given by family members in the Mexican-American group and by family members supplemented by friends or neighbors in the Anglo group. Further, there may well have been a cultural belief operating among the former that a woman should be exempted from usual responsibilities after surgery for a more extended time than may have been believed in the Anglo families. The apparent discrepancy is, at any rate, a matter of more than theoretical interest, since the support system available to the person and the beliefs of those in that system regarding appropriate activities of the convalescent may figure importantly in receptivity to post-hospital instructions.

Cooperation with the physician as another aspect of expected convalescent role behavior seemed to be carried out as well as circumstance permitted. As noted, the restriction on activity was difficult for many, but outright disregard of instructions (which, however, were often related as being minimal—on the order of "take it easy") occured in only two reported instances.

Occasionally, physicians' advice may have aroused cultural sensitivities, but this was reported only once. One Mexican-American woman, who said that she respected her doctor and had good care, was nevertheless irritated with one piece of advice:

> He told me my tissues weren't healing well and I should eat more meat to get protein. Well, what does he think—just because we're Mexican that we eat beans and tortillas all the time?

Nurses did not figure in giving explanation about what to expect in convalescence. When they had taken time in the hospital, however, to sit down and explain what to expect in surgery and in the period afterward, this was remembered with positive regard. One woman remembered with special pleasure that she had been cared for by "a nurse aide or volunteer, I'm not sure which," who had had a hysterectomy herself and "knew how to take care of another person having it." No one could recount any information given them by nurses relative to convalescence. One Mexican-American woman said it would be helpful if nurses could "tell you about the little things—like exercise and diet, and what symptoms to expect—things the doctor doesn't have time to tell you."

An indication of response to lay advice, as opposed to professional advice, was made when respondents were asked whether there was any advice or suggestions from friends or relatives that was helpful to them in convalescence. Such advice was not received or if it had been, was not considered helpful by two-thirds of the Anglo women, whereas only one-fourth of the Mexican-American women said they had not received any helpful lay advice. The "not helpful advice" cited by Anglo women tended to center about the fact that they considered it out-dated. The Mexican-American women who related lay advice usually put it in positive terms of someone who had given them confidence, said not to worry, or cautioned them against doing too much. One young Mexican-American woman said, "My mother's advice was O.K. I might have asked the doctor more if it wasn't for my mother—but then, doctors don't really tell you much."

A general impression that the Anglo women emphasized reliance on professional rather than lay sources was also borne out in the responses to the question, "What advice would you give now to other women having this operation?" Anglo women, more than Mexican-American, tended to stress the importance of having trustworthy professional help and information and the need for a healthy mental attitude. There was a subtle difference in the advice about a healthy mental attitude; the Mexican-American women tended to put it in terms of reassurance, such as, "Don't be afraid," or "Don't worry—

it's not so bad." The Anglo women tended to put it in terms of self-reliance, such as, "Use common sense yourself," "Go into it with an open mind," or "Don't feel sorry for yourself."

DISCUSSION

Although this study focused on differences between the two groups of women, two points need to be emphasized: (1) there were more similarities than differences between the groups; and (2) there was a wide variation in the responses of women within the Mexican-American group. The similarities were evident in the concerns expressed, in the stresses experienced (variations were in the extent of stress, not the types), in the fact that convalescence was the same length of time for each group, and in the matters that "cut across the board" as being helpful—the satisfaction of "having things explained," of having persons interested in one's welfare, of receiving simple warmth and kindness. The differences cited between the groups should, however, alert nurses and other health professionals to areas where additional explanation, support, or awareness of possible cultural sensitivity may be indicated.

The variation within the Mexican-American responses could be characterized as ranging from "traditionalistic" to "typical Anglo." *Traditionalistic responses* could be generalized as stressing family helpfulness, a pragmatic attitude toward the professional, more reliance on lay information, and more open discussion between female relatives than between husband and wife. *Typical Anglo responses* could be generalized as stressing self-reliance, confidence in the professional, skepticism about lay information, and open discussion between husband and wife. Those Mexican-American women who gave traditionalistic responses appeared to reflect a more circumscribed environment where much of their information was from relatives or acquaintances within a neighborhood. They also appeared to reflect a role training that emphasized deferring to the male and being a "whole woman" with the ability to be a satisfactory marriage partner and to bear and raise children. A hysterectomy, when seen as possibly affecting these very important aspects of feminine role, is understandable as creating considerable anxiety. Some of the respondents commented candidly on the effect of male expectations with respect to these matters. One woman said:

> There's something about Mexican men, you know—they want things just right with a woman. Maybe that doesn't apply to French or German or other men, but it does to Mexican men.

Another woman said:

> I think it's mostly the husband's fault—they think about his (the operation) and say the woman's no good. They keep reminding her, "Well, you're no good—you can't have any more children."

In the same vein, another woman said, "Well, they're teasing at first (husbands), but then after a while they get to believe it."

The concern about a hysterectomy affecting feminine role was also evident in the type of lay information prevalent in the Mexican-American communities, or at least selectively attended to; in the concerns that Mexican-American women explicitly expressed; and in actual instances where surgery was delayed because of this worry or because of husbands' reluctance to let the operation be done.

It should be remembered that two-thirds of the Mexican-American women were second-generation so that the probability of a more traditionalistic learning of the feminine role in childhood was high. Information was not obtained on the spouses' generation, but if relatively the same numbers were also of foreign or mixed parentage, then the probability is also high that the cultural concept of masculinity may have been traditionalistic. These notions are strengthened by the fact that this was not a high-income group in which the decline in traditional definition of roles and the importance of some values might be more rapid due to a wider acquaintance with the majority culture.

How persistent the cultural concepts of and attitudes about masculine-feminine roles may be among Mexican-American persons is a question of general interest. These roles are among the first to be learned within the family circle and might thus tend to be persistent through generations. However, role behaviors are modified through interaction with others whose behaviors within similar or complementary roles are different, as in the majority culture where male-female egalitarianism is more pronounced. Actually, the persistence of the traditional Mexican cultural concept of masculinity, which allows little flexibility in the feminine role, is already in doubt among Mexican-American urban families (3). It would appear, however, that it is still an important factor to consider in how Mexican-American women (or other women with similar role training) will respond to situations in which their relationships as women vis-a-vis husbands, or their self-concepts as women able to bear children, are affected even symbolically.

Another question suggested by the results of this study is whether the seemingly greater sensitivity to and awareness of symptoms and reactions that was apparent among many of the Mexican-American women was a response engendered by this particular operation's threat to their feminine role or whether the response might also exist with respect to other illnesses. The question has particular implication for health professionals when they make comparative judgments about how persons (at least women) of Anglo and Mexican descent are responding to any illness or treatment.

NURSING IMPLICATIONS

Because a hysterectomy is a common surgical procedure, nurses may consider the situation from the view of long familiarity; that is, "Oh, she's just having a hysterectomy." For the women in this study, however, it was not "just another operation," although certainly some welcomed it for a variety of reasons. For some, it was not only a major event, but a crisis event in their lives, and as one woman said succinctly, "It's a time when a woman needs a lot of understanding."

As noted, only a few persons mentioned incidents where they were given individual attention related to their own needs above and beyond what would be expected of basic nursing care, and there were no reports of instructions given by nurses relative to convalescence. Perhaps part of the reason for this lack centers around the fact that most nurses see women undergoing this operation during only one phase of the experience—the relatively short time they are hospitalized. They often do not know of the concerns that many women might have had before coming to the hospital or of the difficult decision it was for some and the delay this indecision caused. They may be even less aware of what occurs after the woman leaves the hospital, so that explanations about what to expect during convalescence and reinforcement of physician instructions are omitted simply out of lack of knowledge about the post-hospital period.

Perhaps one of the more important contributions nurses might make, since they are primarily women and since they have the opportunity for frequent contact with the persons in the hospital, would be a tactful finding-out of what the person believes about a hysterectomy. (Obviously if opportunity affords, this is better done well in advance of hospitalization.) Most persons undergoing this procedure are open to any bits of information they hear about it. As noted, Anglo women tend to stress the "legitimate" professional advice, but this is not always true, and for both Anglo and Mexican-American women, considerable anxieties may have been aroused by lay stories they had heard about the after-effects. These lay stories apparently are more pervasive than health professionals might like to believe, and the ones concerning change in feminine role appear especially ubiquitous in Mexican-American communities. The need for continual explanation and support is apparent, as is the need to *not assume* that the person has correct information. Even such basic information as the fact that menstruation would no longer occur was welcomed by at least one woman, who said, "I guess I should have known that, but I didn't."

Mexican-American women may be especially reluctant to ask the physician if he will talk with the husband and explain the operation, yet such a discussion may be one of the most helpful actions that can be carried out. Nurses, of course, may find many informal opportunities to talk with the spouses concerned and to discuss the operation itself and what can be expected afterward. In the more traditional Mexican-American families, however, information from a male physician would be more acceptable, especially that concerning the lack of consequence for sexual relationships and the woman's own "wholeness" as a woman. (One physician routinely and rather effectively injected a note of lightness into what might be a sensitive topic for some by stating, with respect to sexual relationships, "If it was good before, it'll be good afterwards; if it was bad before, it'll be bad afterwards.")

Another implication for nurses and health professionals concerns an aspect of feminine role that seemed to emerge from many of the Mexican-American women's responses. That was the aspect of modesty, but modesty in a deeper sense than simply regard for decencies of behavior. Rather, it seemed more of a feeling that the body is too personal, too much "one's own" to be exposed. A hysterectomy in some sense is an exposure and to reexpose oneself through talking about it could be distasteful—which may have been one reason for some of the (few) women who did not want to be interviewed saying, "I don't like to talk about my operation." An obvious reason for refusal would be (and probably was) the reluctance to talk with strangers, but that does not negate the possibility of the above feelings existing in addition to that reluctance. Some of the comments about dreading pelvic examinations and embarrassment about not being able to get to the bathroom in the hospital seemed a part of this modesty, and so did the unanimous agreement of all Mexican-American women who went home with retention catheters that this was the most difficult part of their convalescence. Catheters with drainage tubes expose to others a very private function.

Certainly this is not to say that Anglo women were not also modest or that they would equably accept exposure of their selves in any sense, only that there seemed to be a quality of modesty which was deeper for many Mexican-American women. It is, at any rate, a factor to which health professionals working with Mexican-American women should be alert.

With respect to the convalescent period, discussion about what to expect could include the fact that the person may feel unduly tired and weak the first day or several days at home, even though she "felt great" in the hospital preceding discharge. She needs to know that driving a car should be refrained from for a while, since especially for those with abdominal hysterectomies, applying the brake can be an uncomfortable and rather difficult action. Of household activities, hanging out clothes and vacuuming may prove to be the most difficult and tiring and should be deferred. Lifting all heavy objects should of course be deferred, and for women with young children at home, the urge to pick them up will be hard to resist. The first shopping trip should be planned as a very short one. Those who have had vaginal hysterectomies need to know that they may continue to have some vaginal discharge and that they should ask their physician about this if he has not already discussed it with them. (Several women found the presence of unanticipated vaginal discharge exceedingly distressing.)

The usual advice regarding marital relationships is that they may be resumed at approximately six to eight weeks, although physicians may vary in their advice on this matter. If an anterior-posterior repair was performed along with a vaginal hysterectomy, the person should know that intercourse may be uncomfortable the first time or two due to the tightening of the vaginal walls, but that this will be temporary.

Discussion regarding the possibility of feeling "blue" and "nervous" at times during convalescence is an area wherein one should tread lightly. There is always the possibility of setting up a self-fulfilling prophecy by leading the person to believe that she can expect these feelings, yet to say that such feelings are nonsense—that no one should feel that way—is unrealistic. Certainly if the woman had wished for additional children, such a statement would not only be unrealistic, but insensitive. As noted, more than half of the women in both groups stated that they had experienced more feelings of nervousness during convalescence than before surgery. Perhaps the best guideline would be to use a simple statement such as, "You might have some feelings of nervousness and even periods of feeling 'blue' but that wouldn't be unusual—some women do." Down-playing concerns about emotional reactions and leading the person to think she is neurotic if she has such responses is a disservice to her. Perhaps male physicians are not always as attuned as they might be to this aspect of the experience and the understanding and acknowledgment by the nurse that the woman's feelings are not unusual will be welcome.

The occurrence of hot flashes when the ovaries have not been removed may be surprising and upsetting. (They do not always occur.) A simple explanation that this may happen because the manipulations involved in the surgical procedure may temporarily disturb the blood supply to the ovaries will be reassuring.

Questions about the length of time required for convalescence cannot, of course, be answered with certainty. The range of time for women in this sample was from two weeks to six months—and may have been more since some persons said they still did not feel recovered at the time of interview. A fairly good estimate would be, however, that the person will most likely be doing many of her usual activities in about a month and undoubtedly will "feel like herself" or even better in about two months (4).

A final implication (and one not confined to nursing) perhaps is so self-evident as to not warrant making. This concerns language. Only two of the Mexican-American women in the main sample were not bilingual, but several apologized for their "poor English." The desirability and necessity of having more personnel in hospitals who are of Mexican descent and/or speak Spanish when such hospitals serve communities with a high Mexican-American population seems obvious. The simple presence of personnel able to speak Spanish is no compensation for lack of other qualities, but understandable and potentially helpful explanations and instructions about both the in-hospital and post-hospital periods are certainly mitigated against by language barriers.

SUMMARY

The experience of undergoing hysterectomy was similar in most respects for both Anglo and Mexican-American women. There were, however, variations that occured in the extent of stress perceived in the preconvalescent and convalescent periods and in convalescent role behavior that appeared to reflect ethnocultural factors. These differences suggest the need to further explore cultural patterning of feminine (and masculine) role as a factor in illness behavior, as well as the need for further comparative studies of illness behavior and convalescent role behavior, and the import of support systems in the latter.

The opportunity and need for nurses, both as women and as health professionals, to provide support and knowledgeable assistance to all women undergoing this common, but major procedure was apparent. Modifications in care based on ethnocultural difference would not need to be extensive in many instances, but could markedly enhance that care.

REFERENCES

1. Williams, Margaret A., "A Comparative Study of Post-Surgical Convalescence Among Women of Two Ethnic Groups: Anglo and Mexican-American." Unpublished Doctoral dissertation, The University of California, Berkeley, 1971.
2. ________________, "________________," in *Communicating Nursing Research*, ed. Marjorie Batey. Boulder, Colorado: WICHE, 1972.
3. Grebler, Leo, Joan W. Moore, and Ralph C. Guzman, *The Mexican-American People.* New York: The Free Press, 1970, p. 363.
4. A useful accompaniment to discussion is the booklet "After Hysterectomy, What." Available from the S. E. Massengill Co., Bristol, Tennessee.

Helping a People to Understand

ANNIE D. WAUNEKA

Wauneka focuses on the public health perspective in nursing. Her work with the Navajo was based on patient teaching from their cultural perspective.

In 1951, my first year on the Navajo Tribal Council, one of the doctors reported on the difficulties of helping Navajo patients with tuberculosis. At that time, although Navajo patients were flown to sanatoriums, some of which were located out of the state, once there, they often refused treatment. Some even walked out in their pajamas and went home by whatever transportation was available. Sometimes, when visiting, parents took their children home with them. This caused quite a disturbance among the health workers and, of course, members of the Tribal Council were concerned that their own sick people were refusing services.

I was appointed by the council to look into this problem and see if I could find a way to convince Navajo patients to remain in the sanatoriums for treatment. It was thought that a woman and mother could better understand their problems.

The doctors had told patients that tuberculosis was carried by a germ that could be transferred from one individual to another through contact. But this idea was not understood by many Navajo, especially those who were uneducated. Even today, out of 100 Navajo people, 85 are illiterate.

It was difficult for me to realize that I would be working among my people on the prevention and treatment of tuberculosis, because I was just as unknowing about the disease as any Navajo on the reservation. I admit that I was definitely afraid to tackle the problem. I told my husband of the appointment and explained what I was supposed to do. He immediately objected saying that I would contract the disease and the rest of the family would get it. We were all afraid of tuberculosis.

I thought about the problem for a long time. I did not know anything about tuberculosis, how to talk about it, whether it really was caused by a germ, or whether the doctors had made up the whole story about "bugs." To explain to other Navajo about tuberculosis, to know what I was talking about, to convince sick Navajo to return to the sanatoriums, I had to find out all about it—what it could do to a human being, where it came from.

I spent a lot of time talking to doctors about it and, over a period of several months, visited the laboratory. I wanted to see with my own eyes what kind of bugs the doctors were talking about. I had to know that there actually were germs.

When I understood enough about tuberculosis, when I learned that tuberculosis could affect not only the lungs but many parts of the body, when I knew I could answer questions, then I was prepared to tell my people that only "white man's medicine" could cure tuberculosis.

But first I spoke to the medicine men on the reservation about what I had learned. In turn, the medicine men explained to me the old Navajo beliefs about what causes illness. It was hard for me, but I had to learn both the old and the new to be able to interpret to the Navajo.

BELIEFS AND CUSTOMS

Today, when a Navajo becomes ill, he must choose between the white man's doctor and his own medicine man. He has to decide which one will cure him. In the past, the Navajo people did not believe in the spread of disease, and this is still true today with a majority of them.

There is no word for "germ" in our language. This makes it hard for the Navajo people to understand sickness, particularly tuberculosis.

I asked the medicine men what they thought caused the lungs to be destroyed; what caused the coughing and the spitting up of blood. According to the stories learned from their ancestors, tuberculosis is caused by lightning. If lightning struck a tree and a person used that tree for firewood or anything, it would make him sick, cause blisters to develop in his throat and abscesses in his lungs. There are other beliefs besides this.

It is difficult for the Navajo people to believe that tuberculosis is not caused by lightning but by a germ that multiplies.

To talk about tuberculosis or health care to a Navajo, one must approach him with courtesy and respect. When we enter a hogan or visit with patients in the sanatoriums, we first talk about each other's relations. This is particularly necessary with the elderly Navajo people. By beginning in this way, we show that we are friendly and interested in the person and have respect for him and that we are, in a fashion, related.

Next we talk about everyday chores, how the family is getting along, whom they visit, how they are making out with the livestock or other sources of income. We ask if they are getting any kind of help. This leads to talk about welfare, sanitation, and, finally, about tuberculosis.

We explain to the whole family how tuberculosis is spread and how the bugs can actually be seen through a microscope. We describe how the sick person starts to lose weight, how he coughs, then starts spitting up blood. We tell about x-rays, that taking them is just like taking a picture of anyone. They usually listen eagerly.

It takes them a long time to answer, because they are thinking about what we have said. They tell us about their family problems and ask who will take care of their loved ones at home, who will look after the sheep and horses if they go to the sanatorium. We discuss these problems and tell them that their families will be taken care of when they go to the sanatorium.

In most cases, it is not necessary to look for help outside the family group, because Navajo families are closely united, and not only in blood lines. They live close by one another. Married daughters, aunts and uncles, and in-laws usually are available to help.

This encouragement we give makes patients less reluctant to go back to the hospital for treatment and cure. It is very hard for the Navajo, especially the older ones who have tuberculosis, to go far from home, because they have never been off the reservation or far from their loved ones.

ADJUSTING TO HOSPITALS

A hospital is totally strange to them—strange people, strange food, strange ways of treating the sick. Bathing facilities, running water, electric lights, and thermometers are all strange.

Among other things, the Navajo do not like to have their persons touched. They do not like someone looking at their bodies without their consent. The Navajo do not like to expose their bodies. Bed rest is also strange to them, particularly if they are at home. They know that they must make a living, take care of the children, take care of the sheep. They do not understand what good it will do to stay in bed and take certain foods and medicine.

All this must be explained. Such foods as vegetables, fish, chicken, or pork are not part of the regular Navajo diet; so this is something else they must learn. The value of these foods must be explained, as well as the value of the drugs and treatment the doctor recommends.

The Navajo does not understand why the doctor in the sanatorium does not come to see him every day the way he does in a general hospital. The patients like to see their x-rays to see if they are "making their way to a cure."

It is the responsibility of the health committee to help the Navajo people understand about diseases, how they are spread, and how they can be prevented. The only way this can be done is through people who are interested and dedicated.

The members of the health committee talk to the doctors in the sanatoriums, so they can explain the progress to the patients. The patient who must stay longer must be encouraged in a way he understands. We explain to him that it will take a lot of effort on his part, as well as on the part of the doctors, to accomplish the cure.

Part of our job is to remind families that patients like to get letters from home, to know about how the children are getting along, and who is looking after the sheep. We tell them that patients like happy letters.

The ones who receive all kinds of complaints from their families want to go home to take care of the problems. When families write such letters, we explain why happy letters are needed.

When patients must be persuaded to return to the sanatorium, we point out what improvement has already been made. The patients admit they feel better in the hospital. They say, too, that they would like to return and will return after the problems at home have been cared for. The health committee emphasizes the danger to the family and how, in the long run, it will be better to be cured of tuberculosis.

It is important to listen to and understand the patient's problems, how he feels about being so far away from home, and just what it means to him to be in the sanatorium.

Another thing that must be clearly explained to the Navajo is that tuberculosis is not a disease peculiar to the Navajo but that it is a world problem, a community disease, and that all health services such as the U.S. Public Health Service are working very hard to stamp out this dreadful disease. We explain that tuberculosis is a disease of long standing and that it is the duty of the Navajo people to help cure themselves.

In the past, the Navajo were not told about tuberculosis in just this way. They were never warned or taught about this disease or that it could be prevented. The only things Navajo patients learned were that, if they were sick, they went to the hospital, got treated, and came home.

I have made films on tuberculosis with the narrative in the Navajo language, which we have shown in many communities. These help to teach the Navajo about tuberculosis, what can be done about this dreadful disease that is killing off our people. The Navajo are interested and active in planned programs throughout the reservation. Through the health committee, they are learning more of what we need to do to raise our children in better health and to safeguard them from disease.

THE BLESSING WAY

When a Navajo patient returns from the sanatorium, a ceremony called "The Blessing Way" is performed. It is a beautiful ceremony performed for those who have been away for months or years, perhaps in the hospital or even in the armed forces. The Blessing Way gives them moral support; it is a happy reunion with a happy spirit. The Navajo knows he is home, that he is welcome, and that he and his family are on a happy journey and wished every prosperity and good health.

I am glad to report that tuberculosis has decreased from first to seventh place as a leading cause of death among the Navajo people. We still have patients who should go to the sanatoriums, who still need to have it explained that tuberculosis is actually caused by a bug discovered by the white man, and that the white man has also discovered the medicine to cure it.

The Navajo patients learn many lessons in the sanatorium and, when they return home, improve their homes because they know that in the hogan with a dirt floor with its uncleanliness, tuberculosis can be developed again. They also bring the message of better health teaching to their families and communities. Now attitudes are changing.

Explanatory Thinking in Chinese Americans

THERESA TSUNG TZU LOUIE

Immigrants to the United States are faced with learning new cultural norms for behavior and new communication patterns for expressing these norms. Usually, the stranger attempts to place his new learning within the context of his old culture, and the result is a unique blend. Louie shows how the Chinese American makes the transition between Chinese and American health belief systems.

The Chinese-American community in San Francisco has more than tripled since the repeal of the immigration exclusion act in 1943. According to the 1970 census, Chinese Americans are the second largest minority group in the city. A gross survey of the downtown Chinatown area revealed that there was one Western hospital serving that population; that the ratio of herbal to Western medical practitioners was 5:7; and that there were an equal number of Western and Chinese drug dispensaries. Herbs were available in grocery stores as well as in herb stores without prescription. The survey also revealed that the Chinatown area had developed a health care delivery subsystem manned largely by Chinese Americans who had been educated in the

An original paper. By persmission of the author.

United States. Many Chinese immigrants, however, utilized public institutions such as the county facilities and (in the case of rare diseases) the University facilities simply because they could not afford private practicioners.

This increase of Chinese immigrants into the Western health care delivery system in the United States prompted the author to study the problems encountered by the immigrant when he is faced with a new, different cultural definition of illness and health maintenance, since how patients define their situation is based upon their specific culture, social interactions, and unique biographical histories. In addition, such a study would advance the knowledge of Western-trained health care professionals who have scant knowledge of the customs and beliefs of herbal practice. Many consider it quackery, and are insensitive to the cultural needs of the patients. Counseling problems are further intensified when the patient does not fully believe in the conventional Western health system, but instead uses an eclectic approach to medical consultation; that is, he uses both Chinese and Western health care systems, either concurrently or alternately.

This paper describes the processes of explanatory thinking, and their culturally related concepts of health and illness, in the Chinese-American illness situation. These processes are believed to be used to "normalize" symptoms. Two basic processes have been isolated: *picking up* and *linking.*

PICKING UP

Picking up is defined as that process in which the individual selectively receives, notes, and retains information from the specific environment. Picking up apparently comes from a variety of sources, such as the recognition of difference in cultures (Chinese versus American); from subcultural differences (professional versus lay); from the mass media (magazines, newspapers, broadcasting systems); from significant others; from the educational processes; and particularly from one's own experiences.

Picking up appears to be cumulative with time, and therefore has an historical aspect. Stories or sayings from relatives are a frequent source of health and illness beliefs that are shaped early in childhood. One women stated:

> We had this remedy from generation to generation. I guess I never asked why. . .we weren't supposed to. We just took it for granted.

Health and illness beliefs can be termed *prepackaged* in relation to the sayings that are passed from generation to generation. Such prepackaging includes a particular formula with foredrawn relationships. An example of a saying is:

> One is born with epilepsy. It is not inherited. They say it's because the mother has eaten lamb during her pregnancy.

There is a ready reservoir of picked up information that may be tapped on call. The content of this information, of course, varies from culture to culture. Concepts, related to the body and concepts related to the care of the body exemplify the reservoir of prepackaged content that has been picked up and retained. The following descriptions are taken from field notes.

Concepts Related to the Body

These concepts include the concept of breath or *hay;* the concept of *blood;* the *hot-cold* concept; and the concept of *foong* or wind.

Hay: (breath, energy or spirit) " Resides in the lung, trachea and heart. One is born with a plentiful [*sic*] or a deficiency of *Hay*. One can take a dietary supplement but it depends on whether the person can tolerate it or not. When a person does not have enough *Hay*, he cannot converse at length or walk a long distance. When a person has sufficient *Hay*, he has strong resistance and does not get sick."

Blood: "A weak person has weak blood. A strong person has stronger blood. He can dispose the poison in him and if the blood moves well illness will not exist. It is like a moving machine. Well oiled machine moves without trouble. When blood does not move well, one has hardened blood vessels and high blood pressure."

Hot-Cold: This concept encompasses the body concept, disease causation symptoms, and food classification. It is the colloquial version of the traditional *yin-yang* concept of the universe. The more assimilated person retains only ideas of some *hot* foods. The person with more traditional ideas classifies symptoms as *hot* or *cold* and uses remedies accordingly to neutralize the excessive effect of *hot* or *cold*. The goal is to reach a balanced state which is health. Disequilibrium results in sickness.

Foong: (wind) "A person gets it by staying at a damp place or being close to a dying person. One knows one has *foong* in the body by the sign of air: bloatedness, bubble in the stool, passing gas, and foam in the sputum." Still-birth creates the worst kind of *foong*. "A woman with a dead fetus carries *foong*. The poisonous *foong* remains in her and is absorbed. She is susceptible to later illness. In the meantime, she may have diarrhea and tummyache."

Two examples from the field notes are descriptive of some of the prepackaged beliefs that recur in the Chinese American. The degree of assimilation into the American culture is clearly indicated.

> "*Yi hay* (hot or cold breath) is usually connected with fried or greasy foods...somehow there is a sore throat involvement. Things that are *liang* (cold or cool) also cause adverse effect. I was never told what it is exactly but its just not good. I just remember my mother saying a lot. And there's nothing you could eat...either it's *yi hay* or *liang*."

> "They say after childbirth the pores are open. So don't wash hands in cold water. In Chinese hospital, you will see husbands bring thermos for their wives to prevent arthritis. They give woman ginger, sour pigs feet, and chicken wine to chase the *foong* out."

Concepts Related to the Care of the Body

These concepts are focused primarily upon a balancing of one's life which maintains the healthy state. Balancing encompasses the concepts of replacement and moderation. Danger is a major concept in relation to the care of the body.

Balancing: The goal of balancing is harmony—an absence of excess. One balances the *hot-cold* status of the body by noting hot or cold symptoms and proceeding to regulate one's diet by selecting the proper categories of food.

Replacement: Balancing requires a codified supplemental regime. Replacement means making up the deficiency which the body is born with or has accrued during the course of life. The expressed purpose is to avoid illness. Foods and herbs for replacement are differentiated according to age, sex, season, and weather.

> "I take *poa chia* (supplemental tea). My father used to drink it Its supposed to be good for bone aches, but mainly for supplement, to build you like vitamins, to keep you from getting sick or catching colds."

Moderation: "Everything in moderation! I guess my parents passed that down to me. I instill some of it to my children...a sense of moderation, but not to the extreme. Don't overdo anything in either direction so you don't throw your system out of balance and that can cause illness."

Danger: The person who is balancing and cautious is concerned with the risk factors. Not only does one follow the codified hot-cold balancing, one is weighing the risks, which some call danger. To be safe, one supplements. To avoid danger, one is quick to define indicators of danger, checking out possibilities of cure, treatment, suffering involved, or prolonged illness.

In addition, to the previously mentioned picking up processes, the final signal that is picked up and noted is the changes that occur in the body signaling a feeling state that is different from one's every day feeling. In other words, symptoms are picked up.

> "Feeling of cold...there is a diminished energy, the head stuffiness and that sort of thing...there's a feeling of depression that you just kind of let go."

> "After my second child, it just hit me. I hurt so much in wrists and joints, that I couldn't do housework."

LINKING

Linking is defined as the process of making connections, of intergrating or creating relationships within oneself. When the individual connects a prepackaged formula with his current circumstances, he is using *integrative linking. Creative linking*, on the other hand, draws a relationship of picked up content to current circumstances with one's own system of logic. Meaning is ascribed to a situation through linking. Certainty, of differing levels, is a result of linking.

Empirical Linking: "Listerine kills germs." The linking of experiential knowledge in which using a mouthwash results in the relief of a sore throat, usually is altered into a level of strong certainty.

Non-Empirical Linking: This form of certainty relates information gained from another's empirical knowledge or through linking past information to future events.

Unfamiliar Information: "I think he says I have a tumor...tumor like bleeding ulcer...I think...Yes cancer is a tumor." Confusion between tumor and ulcer may be a result of linking based upon imagery or phonetics.

Uncertain Information: When uncertain knowledge is linked, the result is doubt. If an individual does not have a tangible source of information to relate to, he will use his own linking.

> "Tumor is a growth. It is like roots spreading over the body. May be it is the nicotine you smoke, going down the intestine and burn a hole there. I think it is something like that. I don't know for sure."

The degree of assimilation into the American culture is frequently determined by the amount of meshing or linking of ideas that have been derived from a variety of sources. In the Chinese American community no pure archetypal forms were found (i.e., Chinese Americans with only Chinese or only American concepts). Instead, there was a great deal of cultural meshing of both Chinese and American concepts.

> "You can get immune to being *yi hay*. Keep on eating fried food and if it doesn't bother you, it won't cause you any trouble."

EXPLANATORY THINKING

Unsystematic, nonrigorous linking of picked up content to a circumstantial situation gives rise to a particular type of causal thinking. Apparently people who have not been socialized in long educational processes exhibit this type of explanatory thinking. Consider the picking-up process described so far; the concept of health and illness is generational and traditional, unquestioned and assumed to be true. The concept of body assumes a natural "born with" view. One's blood, energy, resistence are all predetermined. Nature is closely intertwined with one's health and illness. Temperature, humidity, nature's symbolic referents like *hot*, *cold*, *foong* can all be sources of disease causation. Food can be a source of illness as well as a replacement remedy. The codified content and its determinism result in an "of course" rationale that precludes questioning. The style of imparting sayings, the content of picking up all assume a causal stance. The consequence of linking thus exhibits a posture of totalistic, nonvariant absoluteness, that bears a direct symptoms stamp out in the current situation. This type of causal thinking gives the person a sense of sureness. The illness situation is self-controlled. One is engaged in known remedies and avoids unnecessary anxiety.

IMPLICATIONS

One finds that symbols used to represent illness are drawn from eclectic sources, and are rarely in anatomical or physiological terms. The illness concepts are a bicultural fusion. The theories of illness and remedies are conceived in causal explanatory thinking. Thus, a health practitioner should first familiarize himself with the cultural concepts of health and illness of the population he is serving. He is then in a better position to assess the patient's bicultural illness concept and offer intervention. In dealings with the causal explanatory level of thinking, one must bear in mind the gap between patient's simplistic explanation versus the professional's discretionary thinking. The latter's multivariant explanations divert the patient's energy without relieving symptoms. The patient's concern is mainly symptoms eradication. Explanations to patients must therefore be communicated in a symbolic imagery that is in the patient's reservoir.

In terms of research, it is important to explore the causal explanatory thinking in other cultural groups. There is implication of increased pragmatic application in the client-therapist communication.

Terminal Care at Home in Two Cultures

JEAN FRENCH / DORIS R. SCHWARTZ

Case studies of individual patients are a valuable means for gaining cultural insights; but when these studies are contrasted, as in the following article, our understanding of a particular problem within its cultural context is enhanced. Knowledge about death and dying across cultures would be aided through study of many more individual cases within each minority group, and comparative evaluations of these cases.

Nurses, physicians, and other health workers often fail to recognize how much culture affects the way a patient and his family seek treatment and respond to medical personnel.

It is easy to recognize the barriers to accepting medical care when one is working with a relatively isolated culture. On the cosmopolitan urban American scene, it is often harder to recognize the influence of culture on a patient's behavior.

Two examples from widely separated home care programs of New York Hospital (Cornell University) bear out this observation.

IN A NAVAJO HOGAN

Mary T. was a 59-year-old Navajo woman who was diagnosed as having an epidermoid carcinoma of the cervix. She was admitted to a private hospital for radiation therapy. From there she was transferred to a government (Indian) hospital and was discharged a month later with a poor prognosis. After discharge, she was followed in her home community by the Cornell-Navajo clinic. Here an additional diagnosis of osteoblastic carcinoma was made. She was rehospitalized for 10 days at a mission hospital, but her family wished to give her terminal care at home.

Family members came to the Cornell-Navajo clinic to ask if the staff would help care for Mary after her discharge from the hospital. The clinic physician re-explained the nature of her illness to the family and told them there was no known cure for her condition at this time. The family replied that a Navajo medicine man had given them hope that Mary might be cured and they wanted to seize every opportunity.

The clinic physician agreed with the family about using the "sings" of the medicine man, but asked that simultaneously, with the medicine man's approval, the Cornell clinic staff be permitted to extend whatever help the patient required and could accept.

Mary T. returned to her camp by horse and wagon. The camp consisted of two hogans, the earth-covered lodges of the Navajo, and a sheep corral. One hogan was occupied by the patient and John T., her husband, the other by Mary's niece and the niece's husband. Several nephews, whom the patient had raised, lived in the camp from time to time.

The public health nurse from the clinic and her Navajo aide (the health visitor) made biweekly visits to show the family how to nurse the patient and make her comfortable. When it seemed indicated they gave Mary direct nursing care.

The clinic provided medications, dressings, and necessary equipment. The patient's husband improvised a trapeze, at the nurse's suggestion, so that his wife could alter her position with less pain. Her back had become excoriated while she was hospitalized, and the nurse taught the husband to give back care. He did this so effectively that he was able to halt the development of a decubitus ulcer.

When the nurse checked the supply of medicines on successive visits, however, it became plain that the family was not giving medicine as directed. The Navajo aide believed that the family withheld the pills because they associated the patient's physical decline with the medicines which she had begun to take in the hospital and feared that more would make her worse.

The Navajo people do not distinguish, as most of us do, between health and religious practices. They see health as a perfect balance between man and his environment, an environment that includes people, nature, and the supernatural. We would call this the natural, religious, and social surroundings of a patient. The Navajo believes that illness means that a person has fallen out of his delicate environmental balance and that health can be restored by the acts of a fellowman who has proper and exact knowledge of myth and ritual. That fellowman is the Navajo medicine man and the ceremonies which he performs are known as "sings."

The public health nurse made several visits while the patient was having a sing. On occasions when a sing was interrupted by her visit, the nurse was permitted to give care in the presence of the medicine man.

During the patient's downhill course, the family kept her as comfortable as possible and followed the nurse's suggestion to maintain adequate fluid intake. Shortly before the patient's death, the family called in a native diagnostician, the *ni delnuhi*, who said that the patient would die at noon that day.

The Navajo must burn the hogan in which someone dies, so the patient was moved to an expendable, temporary hogan made of logs and bushes, about 500 yards from the hogan in which she had lived.

The nurse noticed that Mary seemed very cold, although she still responded to sound and movement. John T. had purchased two new woolen blankets and a satin comforter for Mary, and as she became progressively colder, the nurse thought their use seemed indicated. However, the family explained that these new blankets could be used only after death. For the first time, the public health nurse found it difficult to accept the family's ways. By now, Mary was aphasic, her respirations shallow and rapid, but her pulse was still strong.

On the following morning, family members came to the clinic to report that the patient was dying. The physician, public health nurse, and a Navajo aide went out to the hogan and found Mary T.'s condition as it had been on the previous day. The family were taught how to check the patient's pulse and a small mirror was left with them to check her breathing. Later that day the family sent word that Mary had no pulse and that her breath no longer coated the mirror.

NAVAJO DEATH RITUALS

A hogan visit was made to confirm the fact of death. The immediate family and other relatives were gathered outside the temporary hogan.

They asked the nurse if she would prepare the patient for burial. The Navajo are afraid to touch a body after death, because they believe that the spirit or ghost of the departed person is contaminating. Yet the family said that the two nephews could help the nurse and the patient's husband, John, went into the shelter to supervise the activities. It was unusual for a Navajo family to permit Navajos to touch a body, and they later arranged for a cleansing sing to counteract any contamination of the nephews.

When the nurse had completed postmortem care, the husband asked her to dress his wife's body in her best squaw dress, with a long, satin, pleated skirt and a long-sleeved, velvet blouse trimmed with silver coins. A kerchief was put around her neck and her turquoise jewelry—ring, bracelet, and necklace—were put on her body. A clay resembling red ochre was given the nurse to rub on Mary's face to give it a more natural appearance. Her hair was brushed, rolled, and put into a net.

Then John T. took all his money out of his wallet, put it into a little red purse, and had the nurse put this on Mary's body. The squaw blanket was put on her, then the two new woolen blankets, and finally the new satin comforter.

The Navajo aide had been in the temporary shelter during all this time, but the nurse was aware of her reluctance to touch the body and did not ask her to help with the procedure. The husband thanked the nurse for her help and wept when he spoke of what a fine woman Mary T. had been. The family waited outside the hogan for a Christian missionary who was to bring a wooden coffin and officiate at the burial service.

Later that evening, the temporary hogan in which Mary had died was burned, in accordance with Navajo tradition.

IN AN URBAN TENEMENT

Anthony F., a 73-year-old, partly retired junk dealer, who was born in Italy but had lived most of his life in New York City, was discharged from the New York Hospital after a course of radiation therapy following a diagnosis of cancer of the bladder. He had refused consent for an operation, which the doctors thought essential. His several adult children were told of his poor prognosis. Mr. F.'s wife had recently been hospitalized with a myocardial infarction, and was being cared for at home by the youngest, unmarried daughter, Catherine, aged 24.

Since the nursing care of two seriously ill parents seemed more than this daughter could cope with, the hospital staff recommended a nursing home in the vicinity for Mr. F. Both he and the family vigorously resisted this idea.

Six married sons and daughters and Mr. F.'s widowed sister lived in the nieghborhood. They were willing to contribute to the financial support of the F. household and they declared that both parents could be adequately cared for by Catherine.

The home care nurse-coordinator and the social worker both tried to explain how heavy the burden of round-the-clock care would be, but the patients' sons were adamant. Catherine seemed fearful of the responsibility of caring for her father but willing to try. She was able to think about care at home on a tentative and possibly temporary basis. Her brothers were not. So Mr. F. was taken home by ambulance, and the visiting nurse was asked to assess the family's need for assistance and to give what help was acceptable to them. Especially, she would teach Catherine such essential technical procedures as irrigation of her father's indwelling catheter and would help Catherine talk about her own problems.

When the visiting nurse first entered the home, she found Mr. F. sitting in a chair. His catheter had not been irrigated since he left the hospital, although two married sons had been taught to do this before his discharge. Neither the sons nor Catherine were willing to do it now, ostensibly because they were "afraid of contagion." In spite of explanation and reassurance by the nurse and later by the physician, this fear persisted or was used to cover another unexplained reluctance.

This was something the family never really appeared to grasp. They continued to keep the patient's linen and household equipment entirely separate, and his laundry was done at a different time from that of the rest of the family. The only explanation that Catherine could give was that her brothers and her aunt and father wanted it so. Cancer, in this family, was apparently seen as "a plague."

The patient was taught to irrigate the catheter himself, with Catherine willingly bringing and removing the supplies. He learned this procedure quickly. Mr. F. always appeared to be the dominating figure in the home. His orders were quickly carried out by Catherine, who never seemed resentful but, rather, as eager to please as a preschool child.

At first, Mr. F. did very well at home, though his demands were often difficult for Catherine to meet. She had always conformed to the authority of her parents. Throughout the next 11 weeks, Catherine, with the support of the visiting nurse, gave skilled nursing care to both of her parents and tried to remain undisturbed by their increasingly competitive demands for her attention.

Then, as her father's physical condition worsened and his appetite, weight, and strength decreased, he became severely depressed and insisted on almost constant attention from his daughter. The visiting nurse took over more of Mr. F.'s care, but her help was never acceptable to the father, who became dependent on Catherine for his entire physical care and wanted her close by him night and day.

At this point, the patient's wife required rehospitalization as her cardiac condition was increasingly hard to manage. Catherine noticed that although her father was able to retain both food and fluids when she was at his side, he became excessively upset and vomited whenever she left him briefly to visit her mother. He was no longer able to irrigate his own catheter, and since neigher Catherine nor her brothers could accept this task, external drainage was substituted for the indwelling catheter, with the nurse asking herself why an indwelling tube had been considered essential all this time. The sons and daughter still spoke of "contagion" in begging to be relieved of this one responsibility.

PSYCHIATRIC CONSULTATION

Mr. F. now complained constantly of Catherine's inattentiveness, although she was seldom away from his side. She waited on him continually as his condition deteriorated. The conflict between her father's inappropriate demands and her own inability to appease him was so upsetting to Catherine that the nurse requested a psychiatric consultation through the home care program. It is not easy to say whether Catherine or the professional staff found the greatest need for this consultation.

The psychiatrist considered that organic brain disease was responsible for much of Mr. F.'s personality change. As he talked with the family, it became clear that Catherine was the member long since chosen to remain with and care for her parents in their old age and that this decision, made by the family years ago, was looked upon as natural. They saw no reason to question it. Catherine herself had a good deal of hostility toward her parents and siblings and especially toward her father's sister, because of this. Yet she was bound by her training and conscience to fulfill a responsibility, which she could not question.

Unable to take a stand against her own family, Catherine insisted that her father remain at home to die, although alternative plans were again made available. Yet while insisting on caring for him at home, she stated at the same time that she was unable to bear the burden of doing this.

Once the staff fully recognized the neurotic nature of this seemingly simple statement, some of their frustration ended. They began to regard Catherine as a patient who needed their help. During the final weeks of her father's illness, only she could give the physical care that was acceptable to him, but the home care staff, regarding Catherine as their patient, gave her greater medical and nursing support.

During the final week of illness when Mr. F. became unconscious, the visiting nurse took over more and more of his care with Catherine assisting her. Catherine held up well throughout this terminal phase, and her father died quietly at home.

Following his death, Catherine expressed great pride in having been able "to stand it," and gradually settled into an easy and more casual relationship with her sick mother, who was now again in the home. Her mother's needs were complex, but she was far less demanding of Catherine, and both were always able to accept a full measure of the visiting nurse's help.

After her mother's death six months later, Catherine—for the first time in her life—worked outside the home, accepting gainful employment at an unskilled job with enthusiasm. She adjusted well to it and began to make friends among her co-workers.

ACROSS THE BARRIERS

Culture played a part, although only a part, in the behavior of both of these families in a time of terminal illness. One common factor was the extent to which these two families—low on the economic scale by any standards—strapped themselves financially to provide handsomely for the deceased.

Mr. F.'s family went heavily into debt to provide a most elaborate funeral for their father: two carloads of floral wreaths led the procession to the cemetery and this, plus elaborate expense for a handsomely finished coffin, gave great solace to Catherine and her mother, although their own living expenses were sharply curtailed by it during the final months of the mother's life.

John T., providing new woolen blankets and a satin comforter for Mary to be buried in, proscribed their use to warm and comfort her as life ebbed in the expendable brush hogan where she died. After her death, he asked the nurse to place the red purse with all of his money on Mary's body for burial. The turquoise and silver, which represented their family's wealth, was buried with her.

Charon, the boatman, was a familiar figure in ancient Greek mythology, one who ferried souls across the river Styx, to the underworld of Hades. The common custom was to place coins in the mouth of the deceased, so that he would be able to pay his fare across. Neither John T. nor the F. family had ever heard of this myth. Yet both, in the way of their cultures, followed a similar custom, at the cost of providing for the living.

Each family labored earnestly—or at least one member of each family did, with strong approval from the others—to provide care and comfort at home before the death. Each family refused an easier out, institutional care, although this was readily available. Each family accepted medical guidance and welcomed public health nursing care of the sick at home throughout the whole of the terminal experience. Care by the significant helping family member was given tenderly, and professional direction was sought and generally used well.

Yet in each situation, when culture directed otherwise, advice was not accepted. The discontinuation of Mary T.'s medication and Mr. F.'s catheter irrigations represented sharp breaks in care. No amount of teaching, explaining, or requesting could scale the barrier of resistance to these unacceptable procedures and no real understanding of the underlying reasons for the resistance was ever gained.

These two effective interactions show that, even in the absence of full understanding, respect for the family's rights to their own beliefs can enable a nurse to work comfortably and helpfully despite cultural differences.

In most long-term illnesses which are coped with at home, critical incidents will arise which have their roots in the culture of the people. Adair and Deuschle comment:

> One of the greatest problems (in bringing health services) to such people is the refusal—conscious or unconscious—to recognize the peculiar conditions under which (care) must operate. Persons from one culture tend to view another culture in terms of their own. Variations are seen as oddities, to be ignored or reserved for conversational anecdotes and the whole complex of customs and behavior systems peculiar to the other culture is put out of consciousness. . . . In the end, ignorance of these customs and behavior systems results in confusion, inactivity or frustration and the program breaks down because of blocked communication, lack of response or antagonism.[1]

When a public health nurse is giving care to a family whose lifestyle is molded by a different culture, the underlying beliefs which influence behavior can often be identified, either by the giver or the receiver of care. Sometimes they cannot, or at least cannot at the time that nursing is required.

[1] Adair, John, and Deuschle, Kurt. *Personal Communication*, 1970.

We believe that even when the precise explanation cannot be surfaced and validated, respect for the personhood of patient and family makes it possible to continue a relationship that permits the nurse to give care effectively while continuing the search for the cause of the behavior. That respect for personhood we believe to be among the pateint's and the family's rights.

Gypsy Culture and Health Care

GWEN ANDERSON / BRIDGET TIGHE

Gypsies everywhere are nonconformists. They abide by their own cultural rules, at the same time accepting enough of the rules and requirements of their host country to peacefully coexist. Gypsies are also a closed group; they do not accept strangers into their midst easily. As a result, Gypsies are a little-known people and many misunderstandings occur because of that ignorance. The following case study adds to our knowledge of this group and provides clues to more effective nursing interventions.

"Oh no, I didn't go to the hospital to have my babies. I just delivered them in the back of the trailer on the road." These were the words of a Gypsy woman we met while we were taking part in an interdisciplinary study of Gypsies' use of health care services.

Our research team included two medical sociologists, an anthropologist, a public health nursing faculty adviser, a first-year medical student, and ourselves, two graduate students in public health nursing. Our varied interests and abilities proved invaluable and were apparent as soon as we began to collect our preliminary data and review the literature.

Some preliminary data came through interviews with hospital receptionists, doctors, nurses, social workers, policemen, sociologists, and other community members. We were gradually able to piece together a picture of the ways in which the medical community and the general public viewed the Gypsies. Medical people said Gypsies were difficult to work with and unreliable, disregarded hospital regulations about visiting hours and numbers of visitors, were light-fingered with hospital equipment, unconcerned with follow-up care, and inclined to falsify names and addresses. The public saw the Gypsies as a romantic lot of wanderers living by fortune-telling, selling flowers, lying, and stealing.

The literature, though sparse, provided further important background information. We learned that for many centuries Gypsies have consistently avoided being studied and understood by those outside their own culture and have prided themselves on giving the non-Gypsy (Gaje) as little accurate information as possible. Gypsies and their Romany language originally came from India. From there they have traveled to all parts of the world. They have a sophisticated communications system whereby Gypsy communities in any geographic area are in close contact with one another and pass along important information about health, welfare, and legal counsel.

We read of an old legend, which was later repeated by one of the Gypsies in our study, that "it was a Gypsy who stole a nail from Christ's foot at the crucifixion and was rewarded the eternal right for all Gypsies to steal without being caught and punished."

DATA COLLECTION

On the basis of this preliminary information, we all realized it would be impossible to conduct a typical sociological survey of a reasonably sized, random sample of the Gypsy population. The Gypsies were obviously not of a nature to respond to direct questioning from Gajes. Therefore, we developed a research/service plan based primarily on public health nursing visits (by the two graduate students) to Gypsy homes on referral from hospital outpatient departments.

This, however, was easier planned than done, as gaining entry into Gypsy homes was difficult; throughout the entire eight-month study period, we established satisfactory contact with only eight families. Initial home visits to families after hospital referrals led us to false, nonexistent, or recently vacated addresses with no forwarding addresses; phone numbers given the hospital by Gypsy patients also proved false.

We were thus forced to alter our approach and make our initial contacts at the hospital clinics where, fortunately and surprisingly, Gypsy patients faithfully returned for their scheduled appointments. Even so, we and the hospital staff had to do a lot of persuading to convince the patients and their ever-present families of the desirability of home nursing visits and of the need for correct addresses and phone numbers.

Weekly visits were then made at mutually agreed upon times (our Gypsies refused early morning appointments) in the late morning or afternoon. Some Gypsies would move or leave town temporarily, thus interrupting the visits. One family felt that public health nursing services were unnecessary and after three visits requested termination.

We were generally well received (although somewhat warily at first) and were ultimately able to be of service in giving home nursing care, health education, interpretations of medical treatment regimens, and in acting as mediators in Gypsy interactions with the rest of society. We were frequently offered food and drink and were occasionally honored by invitations to holiday or wedding festivities.

Interestingly, the cultural data that our research efforts uncovered were similar to data in the literature. We made many additional health observations, however, in our contact with the eight families. We categorized the observations into "family and social structure," "Gypsy and societal interaction," and "Gypsy health attitudes."

FAMILY AND SOCIAL STRUCTURE

In the first category, which described the family and social structure, we found the Gypsies to be close knit regarding both their families and ethnic units. In all instances, we observed extended families consisting of up to 12 members each per residence, with additional friends and relatives coming and going at will. There was frequent communication among Gypsies via telephone and direct word-of-mouth at frequent informal and formal social gatherings. Our Gypsies loved parties and were encouraged in this by their religion, which recognizes numerous church holiday celebrations. One of the authors was invited to one of the many such religious holidays and was the only Gaje present. Approximately 90 Gypsies within a radius of 100 miles joined in the household singing and feasting on roast pig and spicy, hot, stuffed peppers. The entire party moved on within a few hours to yet another household party, and another, and another still, till the day's end.

This cultural solidarity appears to extend far beyond local or even state boundaries to an almost international awareness among Gypsies of other specific Gypsies in other cities or countries and of ways to reach one another. Gypsy children were discouraged from playing with Gaje children. This is an example of the conscious desire among Gypsies to protect their cultural identity and secrets from Gaje influence and curiosity.

Consequently, although somewhat influenced by the changing times, many Gypsy traditions remain. For example, we learned that Romany is, and is expected to remain, a language of Gypsies alone; that Gypsy law is determined by "the council" and has its own systems of reward and punishment; and that marriage to a Gaje is taboo. In the words of one Gypsy man, "You can never really know and trust a man until you live with him—unless perhaps he is someone like M.D. whose background you can assume."

INTERACTION WITH THE SOCIETY

Gypsy interaction with the society at large is greatly affected by their ethnocentricity, but there are other influences as well. One of these influences is the Gypsy wanderlust, which had taken most of our study families to many parts of the United States and had allowed them to settle down only when forced by illness to remain near medical facilities. Such mobility has greatly interfered with the school enrollment and education of Gypsy children who remain, like their parents, unable to read and write fluently, if at all. As a result of one Gypsy mother's inability to read the directions on a prescription, a topical wart removal preparation was generously applied to the body of her small child with resultant widespread second-degree burns. Our families had many welfare recipients (sign painters are not in demand) and they encountered many associated problems due to prejudices toward Gypsies, their misunderstanding of regulations, changing and false addresses, and written communication difficulties.

HEALTH ATTITUDES

We found that Gypsy interactions with the health care system were not unlike those of other groups in the poverty culture, such as Indians, Puerto Ricans, blacks, and indigent whites. They, too are forced to manipulate the system to receive basic care and often suffer as a result of their lack of sophistication in obtaining the most from the limited facilities available to them. The Gypsies, however, possess a distinct advantage in their mobility, which allows them to shop around for services and in their access to the experiential learning of other Gypsies' past interactions with health care providers.

Our Gypsy families consistently showed a wariness of medical personnel and facilities, and they changed doctors frequently as a result of unfavorable experiences or recommendations from fellow Gypsies. The fact that a certain doctor or hospital had once cured a Gypsy was communicated via the extensive social networks for years after the event had occurred, so that new patients went to previously tested care givers. In one instance, a family traveled to cities in four states nearly halfway across the United States in a futile search for a medical cure for laryngeal cancer, their choices based solely on the Gypsy communication network recommendations.

Where care was satisfactory, the Gypsies remained and trust evolved. However, if a doctor changed a medication without an explanation, or left a promise unfulfilled, or appeared too aloof or impatient, the Gypsies moved on to another doctor in another hospital.

Gypsy health attitudes seemed to fall into two categories: crisis care, which they use predominantly, and preventive and follow-up care, which they use poorly. In crisis situations, where immediate, observable need was present, we discovered a somewhat unrealistic overuse of emergency or clinic facilities. Health was highly valued by the Gypsies and, when illness struck, they demanded the best specialists and offered to pay any price. Whole families were in crisis over one sick member whom they accompanied to, and remained with at, the hospital in defiance of all visiting rules and regulations. Several Gypsies commended a particular hospital for relaxing its visiting hours for them or allowing the husband of a critically ill woman to sleep overnight in her room, or employing a private duty nurse who reported frequently on her patient's condition to the waiting Gypsy encampment in the hospital lobby.

We learned that many Gypsies were aggressively inquisitive, demanding explanations from many health personnel about a diagnosis or treatment. As a result they were surprisingly aware of medical problems relevant to themselves or family members.

A problem we encountered frequently among our families was hypertension and, when we made our weekly visits, not only did all family members gather around and ask to have their blood pressures taken, but friends and other relatives soon began dropping by.

Clinic follow-up appointments were well kept as long as the Gypsies perceived the need. However, when follow-up involved such severe alterations in life-styles as not sleeping late or omitting spicy, greasy foods, it was generally ineffective. One elderly Gypsy woman with diabetes carried all her various pills in one bottle inside her bra. Other Gypsy patients commonly added, omitted, or shared medications with family members. Surprisingly, for such a mobile culture, few families owned automobiles. Most depended on buses or car pools with friends or relatives for trips to hospitals or grocery stores.

Among stationary families, some children were immunized, but this was not so in the transient families. Except for one man who didn't know where to get one, there was no interest in physical examinations. Prenatal care was poor, and eyes went without glasses because of vanity.

DATA ANALYSIS

In analyzing our data, we identified numerous health problems, some uniquely Gypsy and some common to most minority groups in our society, but all with broad implications for medical and nursing care.

To the Gypsies, medicine was for curing, not preventing, disease. Serious problems, such as diabetes and high blood pressure, went undetected until far advanced. Consequently, treatment was often overwhelmingly lengthy and complicated, especially for people who desired immediate results, had limited understanding of disease physiology and pharmacology, and were inadequate in their command of the written English language. The result was mutual frustration and distrust among health personnel and patients as appointments were not kept, as treatment regimens were misunderstood and not explicitly followed, and as Gypsies moved from hospital to hospital in search of help and understanding. In the wake of such confusion, false addresses, and lack of interest in follow-up care, it was practically impossible from a hospital viewpoint to refer, follow-up, and transfer records. Thus, because of their cultural uniqueness, Gypsies overused crisis health facilities and grossly underused preventive and follow-up care resources.

RECOMMENDATIONS

In general, when a Gypsy patient is admitted to a hospital, one way that a nursing care plan can take into consideration the high family-centeredness of the culture would be to have the patient assigned to a room as near the outside door as possible. This will minimize the disturbances caused by many visitors coming and going at odd hours and staying overnight. If possible, highly seasoned, high-fat foods should be included in the patient's diet. If a party can be arranged, it might do much for the patient's mood.

Two other cultural traits we found were a rather high degree of vanity about appearance, particularly facial features, and great female genital modesty. These traits have implications for the need for privacy and for emotional support when treatments are prescribed that involve, for instance, the use of eye glasses or female genitourinary procedures.

Special attention, too, should be given to communications and establishing rapport, particularly in view of the Gypsy distrust of the Gaje.

We concluded that Gypsies were not receiving good, comprehensive, health care partly because of their own cultural idiosyncracies and partly because of inadequacies in the health care delivery system. This is not atypical of minority groups in our society, and once again points out the vital need for health care workers to recognize and incorporate cultural differences in the planning and delivery of comprehensive health care.

A Proposed Diabetic Educational Program for Puerto Ricans in New York City

JOAN BROSNAN

The last two articles in this book were written by graduate students for a seminar in transcultural nursing. Both students were interested in changing one aspect of health care delivery within the cultural contest of their target population. Both examined the current health-care delivery system (the innovating organization) as well as the interaction setting (where the change would occur), and both proposed nursing interventions that take into account the beliefs and values of the patient population. That neither student actually carried out the proposed intervention is not at issue. Instead, the papers are presented as examples of the process of transcultural nursing assessment.

The paper by Brosnan views the diabetic treatment program for Puerto Ricans in New York City within the context of the Puerto Rican value system. She proposes use of the mass media in her intervention. Brosnan's familiarity with her subject led to a lack of literature citation in the body of the paper and a failure to include her data-collection methods. Despite these omissions, however, the creativity of her proposed interventions is a marked departure from the standard nursing assessment and intervention modalities.

An original article. By permission of the author.

INTRODUCTION

According to law, the Puerto Rican is an American. However, the contrast between his rural island, with its Spanish heritage, and the New York metropolis to which he migrates makes him a psychological and cultural foreigner in the city. Puerto Rican migration to New York is estimated at over 40,000 people per year. This migration is a two-way process in which about ten per cent return. Ninety-five per cent of Puerto Rican migrants come to New York City and settle in two main areas: Spanish Harlem in Manhattan and Morrisania in the Bronx. These semighetto areas serve as transition places between Puerto Rico and the United States, containing elements of the culture of each.

The New York Puerto Rican has, in fact, a distinct culture of his own exemplified by differences in the Spanish language from that spoken in Puerto Rico. The Puerto Rican society is class structured and many New York Puerto Ricans prefer to call themselves *Hispanicos* or *Latinos* to distinguish themselves from native Puerto Ricans and recent migrants. Hispanicos classify themselves into three major subgroups.

1. "Los que llevan muchos años aqui" are those who have lived in New York for many years and are considered the core of old residents form Puerto Rico. These old residents are not unattached but live within family groups. Usually grandparents now, they live with or near their married children, their sisters, brothers, or other relatives. More recent migrant kin and friends look to the old migrants for protection, guidance, and advice.
2. "Nacidos y criados" consist of those who have been born or brought up in New York and thus have received all or most of their formal education here. Their education is highly prized and usually this generation speaks fluent English. Men in this subgroup are considered potentially good husbands as they are the most likely to help women in the house. Women, however, are looked upon as less desirable wives since they are said not to be as dedicated to their husbands and children and not to subordinate themselves as much to the demands of their home, as compared to the women in the other groups.
3. "Los que hace poco que estan aqui" are considered to be on the lowest end of the social scale since they do not speak English and lack relatives whom they can rely on in time of need. This paper pertains mainly to this subculture since they are least assimilated into American culture. However,

those who have lived here for many years continue to hold the beliefs and values of their heritage and thus this paper also pertains to an extent to them.

KINSHIP SYSTEM

The center of the Puerto Rican world in New York City is the immediate kinship group. The ideal Hispanic nuclear family is composed of a father, a mother, the unmarried children, and perhaps the mother's mother, who live together in the same household. The nuclear family can also consist of a stable couple without children, a stable couple with their children of prior relationships, one parent with his or her children, or one parent with his or her children and a temporary spouse. Consensual marriages, in which couples live together without having been legally recognized, are less common in New York than in Puerto Rico because New York Puerto Ricans discourage this type of union.

The family is usually split as the father comes to New York first, obtains a job, and then sends for the rest of the family. The father may temporarily stay at his brother's or sister's home or that of a close friend. If the family arrives before the father has obtained an apartment, they too will stay with a relative or friend. They are expected to show their gratitude with gifts of money or goods and by verbal expressions of gratitude.

The father is considered to be the head of the household and his wife is expected to obey and respect his decisions. Men believe women are mentally inferior and have fewer "senses." The father usually goes out by himself and rarely takes his wife with him. If they do go out together, she usually lags behind with some of the children. Shopping for food, and buying clothes, medicines, and personal items for the family is done by the husband.

A family in which strict order is maintained is considered necessary for the development of good children. Boys in the family do have much personal freedom and from the time they are small they are assumed to have an overpowering sex urge or *macho.* Girls are carefully supervised until they are formally engaged since they are considered immanently weak and unwary in protecting themselves from male assault. A high value is placed by Puerto Rican parents on not spoiling their children and on making them obedient. In an anthropological study done by Imogene Cahill, Puerto Rican parents demonstrated less warmth and affection than did parents of other ethnic groups in New York.

The Puerto Rican family unit frequently includes not only the father, mother, and their children, but also aunts and uncles, cousins, grandparents, nieces and nephews. It sometimes includes the couple who sponsor one of the children, the "compadre" and "comadre." If a child is deprived of the care of his parents by death or illness or is abandoned by them, this relative usually takes care of them. Because they are of the same blood, a mother trusts her child to her relative's care without guilt feelings and these children are considered *hijos de crianza* (literally: child of rearing). Old people are given tremendous respect and ritual kin are sometimes considered to be closer than true kin.

HOUSEHOLD ORGANIZATION

Hispanicos consider "living" in a household to consist of sleeping there regularly at night. One may spend the entire day at another relative's house, but one does not live there unless one sleeps there. The basic household unit is the nuclear family, and while other people may live with them, these others are considered to be staying at someone else's home, and are bound by the central authority of the household.

Children who do not live with their own parents may be considered to be either living in their own home or to be staying in someone else's home. The child who grows up without his real parents "in his own home" is considered to be "a child by rearing" and is treated by these "parents" as though he were their own. Children who "live in someone else's home" are not considered part of the family unit.

Certain friends and relatives are considered to be in so close a relationship of trust (*de confianza*) that although they are not members of the household, they may act as they do around their own home. They may thus be seen cooking and washing dishes.

The division of labor inside the household is usually dependent on age and sex. All adult members are expected to work and contribute in some way to the support of the house. The mother or daughter, who works or goes to school, cooks supper and all the women are expected to help in general household work. Women are expected to play a passive role and the ideal wife devotes herself completely to her husband, her children, and her general household duties. Migrant men are not expected to help in households, but their duties in household work usually increase as they stay in New York.

Even in time of need, the migrant is generally reluctant to approach an institution for help. He is accustomed to depending on his relatives or friends whether the problem is unemployment, lack of funds, or illness. Even Puerto Ricans who have been in New York a relatively long time continue to rely on people in their household, although some do learn to seek agency help. In case of medical need there is less reluctance to seek help and more familiarity with New York's institutions, but as a rule the migrant Puerto Rican prefers to have his friends care for him.

THE ECONOMIC SYSTEM

The primary reason for the migration of the Puerto Rican to New York, where ninety-five per cent of Puerto Ricans coming to America stay, is to improve his financial situation. Most of the poor in Puerto Rico work in the cane fields and do not earn much more than $400 per year. A 1950 census taken in a predominatly Puerto Rican section of New York revealed that 67 per cent of the families, where income is pooled in a common purse, earned less than $2,400 per year. Although total wages in New York are higher than in Puerto Rico, unexpected taxes and other deductions are made and real income is not anticipated.

The majority of migrants depend on friends and relatives for an introduction to prospective employers. Puerto Ricans are concentrated in unskilled and semiskilled jobs, mainly in manufacturing and service industries. They are most likely to remain at the level of skill at which they enter the New York labor market. The handiwork jobs available to migrants and the industries in which they are employed are those which are most unstable. Many Puerto Ricans have attempted to escape by establishing small businesses. However, these are the types of businesses which most likely go bankrupt.

Typically, from two to ten families live in places meant for one. Monthly apartment rentals range from $14 to $80 plus utilities. Some rooms in these apartments have no source of ventilation. Often it is up to the tenants to plaster holes in the walls to prevent rats from entering their homes.

CUSTOMS AND VALUES

For recent Puerto Rican migrants the most important and desirable life goals in New York are working hard, acquiring a formal education, and learning English. One is cautious in selecting new friends and tries to maintain the unity and continuity of relationships with one's own family. It is expected that one will help relatives and close friends when they need help. Puerto Rican migrants find, however, that relatives cannot be counted on in New York to the extent necessary. Years of separation weaken relationships to the point that if migrants stay with their kin the latter expect the migrants to pay for their food and rent and encourage them to move out as soon as possible.

Migrants also are shocked to find that New-York-born Puerto Ricans reject identification with recent migrants and often criticize and express dislike for them. It is said in Puerto Rico that men in New York become rascals and shameless because they loose their sense of responsibility towards their wives and children. The women become morally lost because they smoke and drink without remorse.

To obtain one's goals, one may ask God or the saints for help. Dreams or revelations by spirits and ghosts may be a means of foretelling the future—a future over which man has little control. Destiny and chance control the future. According to some medical personnel, "Those Puerto Ricans trust to God more than to instructions." "Our people have faith and hope and believe that God will provide," one Puerto Rican woman stated. "We say, 'Go with God,' and 'If God wills it,' and so forth in speaking of our everyday actions and so perhaps we don't put much faith into man-made rules."

One's dignity is very important and accounts for a Puerto Rican habit of answering yes to a question, whether or not they mean it, so as not to hurt the questioner's feelings. Public health nurses in New York sometimes complain about this saying that Puerto Ricans will listen to their instructions, smile repeatedly, and say, "Yes, yes, I understand"; and then will depart in ignorance, understanding nothing. In general, New York health authorities assume that many of their instructions to Puerto Rican women that are understood will be later vetoed by family councils.

One third of the migrant Puerto Ricans are Negroes. Since their status is higher as a Puerto-Rican-born Negro in this country, the black Puerto Rican is encouraged to maintain his identity rather than try to assimilate into the American culture.

There is a class split amongst New York Puerto Ricans which may be exemplified by the belief that "rich Puerto Ricans make bad employers and pay low wages.' ' Puerto Rican social workers, apparently identified with a higher class, are sometimes said to be unfair to the Puerto Ricans who they are supposed to help. Class feelings are carried over from Puerto Rico where there is widespread antagonism towards the upper class.

In Puerto Rico, it is ordinarily sufficient to divide the day into morning, afternoon, and evening. Hours, minutes, and seconds become important only in a more highly developed industrial civilization. A sophisticated Puerto Rican will ask a continental friend, "Do you mean 5 o'clock Puerto Rican or American time?" Appointments or warnings for visits are not considered necessary. A promise to come does not have to be kept because it is considered a privilege of the relationship to surprise the host with one's visit. People casually drop into one's apartment any time of the day or night.

Puerto Ricans in New York use the radio and newspaper more than they do movies and magazines. Sixty-seven per cent read the *Daily News* and forty-eight per cent read *La Prensa*, a Puerto Rican newspaper. Ninety-eight per cent of all Puerto Rican migrant families listen to the radio. Seventy-seven per cent listen after 6:00 P.M. and over two-thirds of the migrants prefer Spanish radio programs.

BELIEFS ABOUT HEALTH AND ILLNESS

Good health is considered desirable since it permits one to work, and work is a virtue in itself and a means to the future. Beyond man's control, good health is considered a gift from God and sickness a punishment for wrongdoing.

Since New York Puerto Ricans believe that life is subject to fate, one must always be ready for unexpected and intense suffering. Suffering is considered a part of life, especially for the poor, and illness is one form of suffering. When a person develops a chronic illness he wonders what wrong he did for which he is now being punished. An incapacitating chronic illness that cannot be cured, regardless of what is done for it, is considered a fate that one must resign oneself to.

A person may also fall ill because he has done something foolish such as walking in the rain or being careless with mixing "hot" and "cold" foods. One needs to be cautious about eating outside one's home because one can never be sure the food is clean and dirt produces illness. One may also become ill as the result of magic or witchcraft. A person may say that everyone in his family has *achaques* (a multitude of symptoms) when asked about their health, to insure that they are protected from envy. If someone in good health falls ill it may be that someone else envied him and thus cast a spell of *mal de ojo* on him.

If a person becomes ill, he needs to discover the cause before he can be cured, because diseases can have either natural or supernatural causes. Only spiritualists can cure supernaturally caused illnesses. There are certain diseases which affect only Hispanicos which American physicians do not know how to cure.

When a physician is tried and medicine fails to work, it is time to assume that the work is the result of spirits and ghosts. Diseases, especially of internal organs, may be "hot" or "cold" and one needs to take cold medicines for hot diseases. Thus a prescription may not have worked because it violated the rules of hot and cold for that illness. Since medical people may disapprove of or ridicule these beliefs, those who believe in them will not reveal them.

A good doctor or nurse keeps a patient informed as to what is wrong with him, tells him what he must and must not do, and warns him of the consequences. The Puerto Rican patient may continue taking those prescriptions which make him feel better and eliminate those which do not appear to help. If other family members have similar symptoms, they may take some of the medicines prescribed for the one member. Injections are considered to be the most effective kind of medicine while pills are the least effective. Worst of all, however, is no medicine at all. Whenever one is sick one needs to take a purgative in order to throw the disease out of one's body and put herbs in one's food to give him strength.

Although medical exams are considered desirable, personal modesty must be maintained. A good woman does not expose her body nor discuss intimate problems even with a woman unless she has a close personal trusting relationship.

HEALTH PROBLEM CONSIDERED

Extensive diabetic programs exist in New York City Public Health clinics and hospitals which deal with what one needs to teach the diabetic patient so that he will be able to care for himself. These programs, instituted by the middle class Caucasian population, are geared to the middle class American culture. Problems arise, however, when one attempts to teach the Puerto Rican patient about his diabetes in a way in which he will be receptive to taking care of it since he does not have the same cultural orientation as those who are instituting the program. Nursing intervention in this area needs refinement and extension to be effective.

The general life patterns and beliefs of the Puerto Ricans incorporate in them a sense of the powerlessness of the individual. When the Puerto Rican arrives in New York and becomes exposed to a different set of customs, jobs, living conditions, and social organizations, his feelings of powerlessness are intensified, that is, he feels that his own behavior cannot determine the outcome he desires.

Upon arriving in New York, the Puerto Rican migrant depends on others to find a job and living quarters for him. Since many of the jobs held by Puerto Ricans are seasonal, he feels unable to control his economic future no matter how hard he works.

Incorporated into his religious and health concept, the Puerto Rican has a fatalistic attitude towards life. Believing that he has little control over himself, he sees himself subject to the external control of both natural and supernatural events. Predominant reasons for illness are "It is God's Will," or "One has done something foolish and must thus suffer." In either case, the illness is outside of one's sphere of influence.

In dealing with their feelings of powerlessness, Puerto Ricans look to their family and close friends for support. Informal family group councils deal with important matters in which the husband or head of the household makes the decision after listening to the other members. Women, subservient to their husbands, rely heavily on their decision making.

The concept of powerlessness was first proposed by Melvin Seeman who saw it as a significant variable in learning about one's disease. Studying hospitalized tuberculosis patients, Seeman showed that patients who scored above the mean on his Powerlessness Scale scored significantly lower on a test of knowledge about tuberculosis than did a matched sample of patients who scored below the mean. Carrying this concept over to diabetic patients, Padgett looked at the relationship between powerlessness and knowledge of self care. She found that those patients with a higher degree of powerlessness had less knowledge about caring for themselves.

Since a feeling of powerlessness is perpetuated in the Puerto Rican's way of life, it is difficult for him to accept prevention and educational programs in order to gain a mastery over his disease. As a result, more than half of Puerto Rican diabetics are not even reached until avoidable serious complications such as gangrene and diabetic coma occur. To be effective in carrying out a diabetic educational program among Puerto Ricans, it is essential to consider the influence of powerlessness on the diabetic patient and plan interventions accordingly.

PROPOSED INTERVENTIONS

Just as medical people entering a foreign land need to be educated about the people they are to deal with, New York City medical personnel need to be educated about the Puerto Rican culture to be effective in working with them. Since it has been pointed out by Puerto Ricans that many New York medical personnel are prejudiced against them and that sometimes upper-class Puerto Ricans treat them with less dignity than a stranger would, an initial job qualification needs to be a receptive attitude towards the culture. A fluent knowledge of the Spanish language is desirable but not essential since there is always someone in the area who can act as an interpreter. A one week intensified in-service educational program for public health nurses, which deals with the Puerto Rican culture, the changes it is going through, and the special methods of intervention required, needs to be set up. A public health nurse-clinician should be hired in each public health district so that she can advise the public health nurse who encounters difficult situations or problems.

Since over one-half the diabetic cases remain undetected until complications occur, first the Puerto Rican needs to be educated about diabetic symptoms. The hypochondriacal attitude prevalent in the Puerto Rican culture will be an asset in this area. In the *Daily News* and *La Prensa*, the two most widely read papers among the New York Puerto Ricans, educative articles concerning diabetes should be printed. This information should also be broadcast over radio after 6:00 P.M. on Spanish speaking stations. A friendly woman's voice should announce where the clinic is and how to reach it, since this will be less threatening to the Puerto Rican woman and probably will be more acceptable to the Puerto Rican man. The woman announcer should speak at a personal level and extend the invitation: "If you wish to visit, an appointment is not necessary and we will be glad to see you anytime during the day or evening." Both she and the newspaper article should emphasize that it is God's will and fate that they are either listening to the program or reading the article so that they will come in for a checkup, especially if they have any of the symptoms mentioned or if any of their relatives have diabetes.

Since Puerto Ricans are fearful of public organizations, the public health nurse will still have to go out into the Puerto Rican community to make initial contact. This nurse will be assigned to her own specific area within her public health district. Since there are not enough public health nurses to visit each family, a random sample of homes will be visited initially. Since evening is the time when most of the members of the household are at home, she will make her visits at this time. On her first visit she will try to establish herself as an interested friend of the household and will not attempt to advocate any public health measures unless asked.

During her next visit, she will begin talking with the family about her ability to control diabetes when it occurs. She should explain in a simplified manner the nature of the disease and how it can worsen unless she or the public health clinic brings it under control. She will explain that it can cause harm to them unless she can bring it under control before they are even aware that they have it. Then she can propose that she has a method, a test, to see if they have diabetes and she would like to let them see how she does this. Explaining that she will need to use their urine, she will ask them each to take one of the urine cups that she has with her and after voiding in it give it back to her. Testing the urine with her clinitest and acetest tablets, the public health nurse can let the family observe it's strange effect. She can ask them to tell their friends and neighbors about her so that they too can have their urine tested.

Upon obtaining a positive result, she will tell the person in question that it is possible that he has the disease but she needs to make some further tests to be sure. To do this, he must come to the clinic with her and see a doctor. Since the clinic will be open in the evening until 11:00 P.M., he can go back with her after she has finished her visit.

Whether the person originally came to the clinic himself or whether he was contacted by the nurse as a result of a home visit, upon positively establishing that the person in question has diabetes, the nurse will visit the home in the evening and propose a family meeting. Because the Puerto Rican looks to his family for support, the nurse can present the family with the patient's disease as their problem and her problem, stating that she is going to work to control it with them.

In evening sessions, she will teach the family more about the disease and will try to elicit active participation from them. She will convey to the family the idea that it is the will of God that she is here. If the person whom she is dealing with is religious, she will encourage him to pray to God for obtaining all her knowledge to be able to control his diabetes.

Because she realizes that the Puerto Ricans will answer yes to a question out of politeness, the nurse will avoid asking questions with "yes" or "no" answers such as "Do you understand?" Instead she will ask questions such as: "What would __________ (patient with diabetes) do if he feels nervous, weak, sweaty, and very hungry?"

The nurse can stress that it is the will of God that they know what to do when this happens. However, if they do forget or have a diabetic problem which they can not deal with, fate has set up a special telephone number for them at the clinic. They must carry this number with them at all times and are to call at any time of the day or night when they do have a problem.

In planning his diabetic menu with him, the nurse will encourage the person to use herbs from the spiritualist and to only eat all hot or all cold foods at one time. Familiar with Puerto Rican foods, she will tell him which foods are taboo for him and will help him set up menus based on his regular food habits. She may encourage him to take an occasional purgative if he feels that this will be beneficial.

Since Puerto Ricans are very receptive to getting injections and thus the magical powers of the injections, the public health nurse will probably not encounter many difficulties in teaching the patient about his injection. However, she must warn the patient and the rest of the family that it is trictly taboo for anyone else to touch his medicine since it was made to be beneficial only to him and will harm others.

The public health nurse can tell the patient that fate will give him certain warnings that he must go to the clinic immediately. These will include such things as open sores or infections. Since fate has sent the public health people to take care of him, if he develops a toothache and goes to the dentist, the dentist needs to know that he has diabetes and is being controlled by __________ Public Health Clinic. This dentist must first contact his clinic before he treats him.

PREDICTED OUTCOME

This plan of action should be proposed to the New York City Public Health Department. Possible initial increased costs due to the public health nurse orientation program, advertising through public media, and the extended hours of service would eventually be more than offset by the decrease in costs to the city hospitals because fewer diabetic patients would be hospitalized with complications. The New York City Welfare Department would also benefit since fewer people who have diabetes will become incapacitated.

Because the diabetic program would be viewed as God's Will and Fate that they come into contact with this public health nurse, the Puerto Rican should be more receptive to learning about and caring for his diabetes. By having the same public health nurse work with the family and encouraging friendship on a personal level, the feeling of alienation of the Puerto Rican to public agencies would decrease and thus Puerto Ricans would be more receptive to obtaining treatment for other ills. Knowing that there is a "Help Line" available to him at any hour, the Puerto Rican diabetic will feel comforted by the fact that there is outside power to help him deal with a situation in which he feels he has lost control.

Having the public health nurse make evening visits increases the chances of her being accepted by the family, including the head of the household, since they will come to know her personally rather than hear about her from the one member receiving care. They will also be more likely to become more involved with the patient's illness and thus be more apt to give him support and encouragement. The evening is also a good time for case-finding because other people are around at that time.

By respecting and encouraging Puerto Rican beliefs that do not interfere with health practices, the nurse conveys an accepting attitude and shows that she respects them. The trust relationships which she thus builds up will make the Puerto Rican more receptive to her medical beliefs and more apt to continue to follow them.

EVALUATION

An increase in the amount of Puerto Rican diabetics attending or receiving services from the Public Health Department, and a decrease in the amount of diabetics being admitted to hospitals with complications due to their diabetes would indicate receptiveness to this diabetic program. Statistics of the number of cases in these two categories should be computed before the initial onset of the program and then in two years. The results would indicate the program's effectiveness.

REFERENCES

Beuma, John, *Spanish Speaking Groups in the U.S.* Durham, N.C.: Duke University Press, 1954, pp. 156-89.

Cahill, Imogene, "The Mother From the Slum Neighborhood," Conference on Maternal and Child Care. Ohio: Ross Laboratories, 1964.

Cole, Mary, *Summer in the City*. New York: Kennedy and Sons, 1968.

Dooley, Eliza, *Puerto Rican Cookbook*. Virginia: Dietz Press Inc., 1950.

Handlin, Oscar, *The Newcomers*. Cambridge, Mass.: Harvard University Press, 1959.

Landy, David, *Tropical Childhood*. New York: Harper & Row, Publishers, 1959.

Lewis, Oscar, *La Vida*. New York: Random House, Inc., 1966.

Mills, Charles Wright, Clarence Senior and Rose Kohn Goldsen, et al., *The Puerto Rican Journey*. New York: Harper & Brothers Publishers, 1950.

Padilla, Elena, *Up From Puerto Rico*. New York: Columbia University Press, 1958.

Rand, Christopher, *The Puerto Ricans*. New York: Oxford University Press, 1958.

Seeman, Melvin, and John Evans, "Alienation and Learning in a Hospital Setting," *American Sociological Review* 27, No. 6 (1963).

Sexton, Patricia, *Spanish Harlem*. New York: Harper & Row, Publishers, 1965.

A Proposed Tuberculosis Treatment Program for Papago Indians

MARY C. WINN

Like Brosnan, Winn chose a population with whom she had once worked, and placed her nursing process within public health. Unlike Brosnan, Winn is concerned with secondary and tertiary prevention. Clearly and concisely written, this paper is a model for assessment of the cultural context of nursing.

CONTEMPORARY PAPAGO CULTURE

Introduction

The Papago Indians are members of the Piman subgroup of the Uto-Aztecan linguistic stock. They number approximately 12,000, and primarily reside in southern Arizona. About one-half this number reside on one of three federal reservations: Sells, San Xavier, and Gila Bend; most of the remainder are distributed among neighboring communities.

The present reservation land is also the traditional land of the Papago. It includes the area between the Gila and Santa Cruz Rivers, west to the Growler Mountains, and south to the Mexican state of

An original article. By permission of the author.

Sonora. The land is hot and barren, characterized by wide valleys and rugged mountains. Rainfall is seasonal and generally low, 5 to 15 inches depending upon the elevation. Streams are intermittent; the only permanent source of water is provided by mountain springs.

During the seventeenth and early eighteenth centuries the Papago had intermittent contact with the Spanish. During this period wheat, cattle, and some fruit trees were introduced and added to the basic diet of beans, corn, and squash. All food was grown by flood farming methods. In addition to farming the Papago gathered wild plants and seed and hunted for desert rodents and small animals.

A further source of change resulted from periodic Apache raids. For more than 150 years, beginning in the 1690s, Apache raiding parties pillaged and terrorized villages in the Papago territory. The activity of the Apache was perhaps the single most important factor in altering the geographic distribution of the various Piman groups, and is reflected in the location and relationship of present Papago villages. Prior to the period of Apache raiding, the Papago had lived in many small and widely dispersed villages. These included summer residences in the valleys, where the crops were planted at the mouth of washes, and winter homes in mountain villages near permanent sources of water. As the threat of the Apache became greater, dispersal in small groups was no longer possible (Spicer, 1949) and the Papago were forced into a small number of larger defense villages. The situation persisted for almost 200 years until the Apache were finally subdued by the U.S, Army, after the Gadsden Purchase in 1854 brought the area under the jurisdiction of the United States.

After the pressure of Apache raids was removed the Papago again dispersed and new villages were established. Villages derived from former defense villages were in close geographical proximity and maintained their cultural ties. According to Hoover (1935), the present day Papago villages can be traced to about twelve common centers that existed before 1860. Each of these represents a tribe which, spreading from a main village or pair of villages, has established new communities. Underhill (1939) recognizes the same group of ancestral defense villages and calls the offshoots of the original villages "daughter villages." These village areas coincide fairly well with the larger units of plains or drainage basins, imperfectly set apart by mountain ranges.

Social Organization

According to Underhill (1939), the Papago were originally divided into two patrilineal moieties and five or six patrilineal sibs. Neither moiety nor sib associations appear to affect the choice of mates; the only function of these groups is ceremonial. The kinship structure is is bilateral with no greater emphasis on paternal relatives than on maternal ones. Marriage is theoretically restricted between all relatives as close as third cousins, but in practice the degree of relationship may not be very carefully reckoned. From an analysis of Papago matings Zimmerly (1968) reports that village endogamy seemed to be the rule with a trend, through time, toward village exogamy.

The nuclear family is a meaningful Papago social unit that exists as one among a number of other relatively contiguous nuclear households made up of relatives. Kinship can be traced to many individuals in one's village or beyond and domestic life and cooperation within this network of relatives takes many forms. Papagos speak of their obligations to relatives, relate meaningful experiences with them, and even lump classes of them together terminologically; but the nuclear household residence is a vital element in the socialization of individuals. The structure of kinship villages and their ecological relationships persist from the aboriginal culture and provide a Papago individual with a social environment that is completely oriented to interactions with relatives of varying degrees of genealogical closeness (Waddell, 1969).

The Papago family continues to be patriarchal and there is always a recognized head of the house. Most often a household, on the reservation or in some of the rural farm communities, will consist of the old parents, unmarried children, and married sons and their families. Since relatives may be depended upon for hospitality, it is a rare household that does not also include a widowed daughter, a distant cousin, or a child whose parents have died or remarried. Brothers or sisters of the old parents, also regarded as grandparents by their siblings' grandchildren, may also be a part of the family. All of these individuals are not necessarily residing in the home at the same time. There is movement on and off the reservation as seasonal wage work is sought. However, at all times the patriarchal household serves as a home base for the family members.

In a typical household of three generations, the grandfather holds authority over the group, and each married son is head of his own family. If the grandfather grows too old for active responsibility his authority passes gradually into the hands of the son who is generally considered to be the ablest, not necessarily the oldest. Although the head of the house always has the final word, he has a strong obligation to solicit the opinions of all the other family members before the final decisions are made. Even small children are consulted in things which concern them directly, and a child's decision as to whether he wishes to go to school or the hospital is seldom questioned.

Seniority and respect for elders is the most important guideline for personal relations in the household. The child not only respects his parents, but he must also defer to older brothers and sisters. Each person in the family seems to have some authority over all those younger than himself. Men, as a rule, have greater prestige and authority than women. Descent is reckoned through the male line and inheritance is from the father. Older brothers have more authority than older sisters, and all boys expect their sisters to wait upon them in the home. Men usually receive and spend the family's cash income. Even if a woman has a strong personality and actually makes decisions the man is always the family spokesman, and the woman will disclaim authority, at least in public. However, women are not relegated to an inferior position. They are never ordered about and are never servile toward the men. The attitude of both sexes is simply that their duties and spheres of authority and influence are different.

The typical Papago family household is composed of a small cluster of adobe buildings in a clearing or in a part of a larger village settlement with the clusters scattered widely. Off the reservation in the farm camps a similar arrangement is used. The cluster consists of a permanent nucleus of one or more nuclear or extended families attached to the encampment the year around. There is a seasonal enlargement of the encampment during the height of the season when reservation relatives move into the adjacent buildings on a temporary basis.

The main house is sometimes one room, but more often there may be several rooms, or, if the family is large, several small houses. Nearby is the ramada, roofed with dry grass and often protected on two or three sides by upright octillo branches. In good weather all cooking and household chores are done here. One or more tiny huts serve as storerooms.

Village Organization

The three reservations number eleven village units whose location has changed very little in the 200 and more years since Kino visited them. The reason is obvious. They were located in spots which were then, as now, the best for cultivation. The eleven village units form the outstanding divisions in Papago country and the loyality of each individual is above all else to his village and its partners (Underhill, 1939). Jones (1969) recently studied subdivisions of the population. He also suggested eleven village groups based on dialect, marriage patterns, competition in sports and games, cattle roundup areas, cactus groves, and well-site utilization. His village units also correspond closely to political districts. Apparently, the Papago have had relatively little movement of village location in the 100 years since the ending of Apache raids.

With its officers and activities each village functions as a political entity. A headman acts for the villagers in outside contacts, especially with non-Papagos. He may inherit office or may be elected by the village council, but he holds office only by common consent. He may be replaced at anytime his work becomes unsatisfactory. He is a spokesman rather than a leader, expressing village attitudes rather than forming them. The more accurately he reflects the opinions in his village the better he is at his job. No Papago tries to make himself a "big shot." However, a headman may be powerful. Remarkably foresighted, concerned with his people's welfare, he is responsible for them and is expected to feel his responsibility. Therefore, although he may not formulate opinion, he guides and helps it along. He calls the meetings of the village council, composed of all the adult men, to talk over decisions of any importance. A headman does not act on important matters until his council agrees on the course. Unanimity is a strong Papago idea—one they usually achieve at the cost of speedy action. Some issues, never agreed upon, are never acted upon; and when outsiders demand fast action, not allowing time for unanimity, Papagos are disturbed.

Indian villages off the reservation have informal leaders who are usually the eldest and most prestigious individuals. In addition, there are elected leaders, frequently younger men, responsible for organizing village events and dealing with representatives of the Indian Bureau or other Anglo institutions.

Tribal Council

The Papago had no history of any type of tribal organization. Before their contact with Anglo-American governmental methods, each village was autonomous. In 1935, the reservation was divided into political districts derived from both dialect and defense village ancestry (Hackenberg, 1964). The tribal government is now organized around these districts, each with its own council composed of representatives from the various villages, apportioned on a population basis. Each district council sends two representatives to the tribal council (Jones, 1962). There was no immediate acceptance of tribal organization in the terms in which the government saw it. There never had been a subordination of one village group's interest to another, nor was there now. Representatives were not regarded by their districts as empowered to enact legislature but were thought of as "legs," to use the old Papago term; that is, messengers and communicators of news to their district councils (Spicer, 1962). Until 1956 the tribal franchise was restricted to adult males; at the tribal elections in the spring of that year, women voted for the first time. As women become more independent through off-reservation work they are playing an increasingly important part in tribal government.

Following the old pattern or respect for the old, when the tribal council was established the Papago elected their elderly headmen to the council, as a result the younger English speaking men have not found as much scope for their talent and ambition on the reservation as they have off. Even as the composition of the council changed over the years and younger men were elected to serve as council members, the pressure of tradition still limited their influence on the council.

Values

Many of the old values continue to operate in present day Papago culture. Responsibility and subordination to the will of the group is taught from early childhood. Avoidance of quarrels is stressed. The peaceable man or woman is admired. Personal achievement directed toward ostentatious self-gain is severely criticized. The person who is outstanding in any way is expected to maintain a modesty about his accomplishments.

Papagos have always been workers and they readily accepted the paid work offered by the government and the surrounding communities. A temporary migration to work for pay had been an old expedient of the Papago to eke out their subsistence. Families had been gone for a few weeks, individuals for a whole winter, their pay being their food while working and some trade goods or food to take home to the family. Money pay has affected the reciprocal network extending to distant relations. It is easily concealed so that anyone so tempted can fail to contribute to the family support. An economy of abundance was changed by wage labor to an economy of scarcity. It has meant the substitution of investment by saving for investment by giving. This substitution, however, has been incomplete and many Papago continue to contribute what they have to any relative who is in need.

A good man in the Papago sense is a useful member of the group, peaceable and loyal. He is industrious so that others will not have to support him and generous with what he has.

Drinking in Papago culture has stemmed from a ritual-social context and carries with it the power to affirm affections and to seal friendships. Drinking is not disapproved of even if it occasionally leads to difficulties with legal authorities, although inappropriate excess may be frowned upon by other Papagos (Waddell, 1969).

Beliefs about Sickness

Many Papagos still believe that sickness comes from offending one of the many supernatural forces which menace humans. The ghosts of the dead are still believed to bring sickness, returning as owls or other animals, usually at night. Because of this Papagos are very reluctant to mention the dead by name and may refuse to answer questions concerning cause of death in family members. All animals are endowed with supernatural power which they can use to send sickness. This possibility, together with the fact that it may be a ghost, makes any animal a potential threat, and thus the Papago take great care not to offend animals.

Illness can also be brought on by thinking evil thoughts. The great emphasis placed by Papagos on peaceful living and their avoidance of quarreling has already been mentioned. A Papago is constantly reminded that the kinds of thoughts that cause quarrels may also cause illness.

If, despite all precautions, a Papago becomes ill, he may go to a medicine man or *makai* to find out what caused it. The Papago makai is a diagnostician and not a curer. Through the use of rock crystals or other ritual objects the medicine man will determine what supernatural force has sent the illness and indicate which "singer" can cure it. If an animal has been offended the medicine man knows which singer has the power, through songs and fetish, to placate the animal. Sometimes the medicine man will diagnose an illness as a "white man's" sickness for which a doctor should be consulted. The Anglo doctor is most likely to be consulted for sudden acute illnesses which will respond in a short time to medication. More women (than men), particularily those close to the Indian Hospital at Sells or one of the public health clinics, seek Anglo medical attention for their children and for themselves. Men seem more conservative in this area and are slower to use the available Anglo medical facilities.

Many Papagos, especially those living in the northern and western districts, are still not convinced of the superiority of modern medicine and many use either the medicine man or the clinic, depending upon how they have diagnosed their illness, i.e., as an Indian sickness or as a White-man's illness.

HEALTH PROBLEM

Introduction

Southwestern American Indians, including the Papago, often differ significantly from the Anglo population in the frequency, distribution and manifestations of disease. For the purpose of this paper, attention will be focused upon one particular problem, that of tuberculosis. Sievers (1966) states that tuberculosis is the foremost cause of obscure illness in the Indian population. The presence of the disease is sometimes inapparent. In particular, extrapulmonary tuberculosis often has the unrecognized capacity to mimic other diseases. Furthermore, since the onset of tuberculosis is generally undramatic, the tendency is to seek a cure from native medicines, the medicine man, and/or the herbalist before turning to the Anglo physician. Many Papago are diagnosed as having tuberculosis for the first time when they seek off-reservation employment and have an employment physical examination. Another means of detection is hospitalization for some other reason, the admission chest film often showing quite extensive pulmonary tuberculosis.

Present Method of Treatment

Hospitalization for the treatment of tuberculosis has not been too successful for the Papago patient. Approximately fifty per cent of the Indians hospitalized left the hospital before their treatment was completed. Of these, perhaps twenty to forty per cent take their medication irregularly or discontinue it altogether (Fox, 1962). Successful treatment of tuberculosis requires a minimum of two years of chemotherapy and premature interruption of medication leads to a high risk of relapse. If patients can be kept in the hospital, the staff can make certain that they take their medications. However, to keep the Indian patient in the hospital isolated from his family for six to nine months solely to insure that he takes his medication is extremely difficult if not almost impossible.

Hospitalization has proven unsuccessful for a number of reasons. One of the major factors is the separation from family and friends. Good medical care from the Papago's point of view requires that the patient be treated for almost any condition at home by relatives, friends, and medicine men who provide emotional support as well as technical skills required in treatment. In time of sickness he expects his family to surround and comfort him. At the same time, family members feel obligated to remain close to the patient, to take charge of his treatment, and to reassure him as to his place in, and importance to the family group.

At the present time, the Papago who is diagnosed as having tuberculosis is hospitalized off the reservation, either in a Veteran's Administration Hospital, if he is eligible, or in a hospital operated by the Indian Health Service. Both hospitals are located in Tucson, Arizona. Geographical distance makes it difficult for family members to visit. When they can visit they must do so at the convenience of the hospital and not when they are free to come. In addition to physical separation from family, the Papago is among strangers, whether Anglos or Indians from other tribes. In either case these other patients are not members of his family group, and they are not persons from whom he can expect to receive psychological support during a period of stress.

Added to the stress of separation is the Papago's fear of the dead. As has been mentioned, many Papago still fear the ghosts of the dead.

In the aboriginal culture, immediately after a death, the family pulled down the house of the deceased to prevent its being visited by ghosts. Even those Papagos who have had extensive contact with Anglo institutions, such as schools and off-reservation jobs, maintain a strong adherence to the aboriginal cultural system. Consciously they may agree that hospitals are safe places and necessary for treatment, subconsciously they react to them as dangerous places inhabited by the ghosts of strangers.

Many of the older Papago still remember and believe the old teachings regarding the malignant effects of being in the presence of a menstruating woman. The touch of a menstruating woman can weaken a man. In the Anglo hospitals where most of the care is given by women, how can the patient be certain that the Anglo women know proper behavior during their dangerous period? How can a person get well when unclean women are touching you and draining your strength? The feat of this has caused many older patients to leave the hospital before completion of their treatments.

These are a few of the factors that interfere with successful hospitalization for tuberculosis. Some are more influential than others, but these and other values that conflict with Anglo medical practices contribute to the high per cent of irregular discharges for Papagos being treated in a hospital setting for tuberculosis.

This writer proposes that the approach to the treatment and control of tuberculosis among the Papagos be changed. This change would be made in two areas, the hospital where treatment is initiated, and the public health clinics where the continuing treatment and follow-up care is received.

Proposed Changes

When hospitalization becomes necessary the individual should be prepared before he is admitted to the institution. Preparation will begin in the home with an Indian Health Service nurse working with and through a tribal community health representative. The total family will be included in the discussions since the individual concerned will be greatly influenced by the opinions of the entire family group. The final decision to enter the hospital will be left to the individual; however, group concensus is an important factor in determining whether or not the individual will accept hospitalization. If hospitalization is reserved for those patients who are physically too ill to be able to be up and about, for patients with complications and emergencies, or for those with a concomitant disease, acceptance of the necessity for it will be more easily obtained.

Once the individual decides to accept hospitalization, arrangements will be made to admit him to the hospital nearest to his home.

If it should be necessary to hospitalize the individual at a distance from his home, the hospital nurse coordinator working with the Indian Health nurse and social worker will arrange for a family member to accompany the patient and be housed close to the hospital. This family member would have free access to the patient and through the cooperation of the ward nursing staff would be involved in the nursing care of patient.

Hospitalization when possible should be limited to four weeks. The rationale for the four-week period lies in the magical properties of the number four. Things done four times, songs sung four times, are an integral part of any Papago ceremony. By using deeply ingrained folk ideas of curing practices, greater cooperation with the medical program can be obtained.

Something could also be gained by granting to the medicine man the same privileges and respect that the hospital now gives to the priest and minister. The medicine man's usefulness need not stop at lending passive approval to the medical program. A medicine man who is allowed to conduct a curing ceremony in the hospital may be of assistance in persuading a patient to remain in the hospital until discharged.

Following this brief period of hospitalization this writer proposes that the Papago patient be discharged to his home community for follow-up care and supervision. This care would be given by the tribal community health representative, who would function under the supervision of the local Indian Health Service nurse. The same arrangement would be used for those patients not hospitalized or who decide not to be hospitalized.

Studies in Madras India have shown that if patients took their drugs as prescribed, success rates were similar whether they were treated in the hospital or at home. The same studies also showed that most patients had already infected their household contacts by the time they were diagnosed. This means that by the time patients present themselves for treatment, they will have already infected most of their family members who are going to catch tuberculosis from them; thus there is little further danger in keeping them up and about as outpatients (Moulding, 1967). Similar studies have been conducted in Scotland and England with comparable results. There is no reason to believe that any different results would be obtained if outpatient treatment were substituted for hospitalization in the treatment of the Papago who has tuberculosis.

The tribal health representative mentioned above is an individual who is a member of the tribal community he serves. He resides within his own community, and his training and orientation, though identified with health, are much broader in scope. He functions as a liaison person who identifies with his tribe and interprets to them and to the outside world their needs for the purpose of bringing existing health resources to bear upon their health difficulties. He also translates the advice of the health professional to Indian people in such a way that it is more clearly understood and a greater impact is realized from the health professional's efforts.

The community health representative is selected for those traits and characteristics which the tribe feels he must possess in order to function effectively, within both the Indian and the non-Indian community. The personal characteristics that are emphasized are a sensitivity and ability to recognize the needs of the community; an awareness of prevailing attitudes, beliefs, and practices related to health; and the ability to communicate information to both the Indian and the non-Indian community.

The community health representatives have had specialized training in home nursing, environmental health, and advanced first aid, and have been functioning on some of the reservations since 1969. This writer is proposing that their use should be broadened to include the care and supervision of the patient with tuberculosis.

Since the tribal health representative resides in the community, the chest clinic facilities will be readily available to the local residents. One special day each month, or one special afternoon each week, would be set aside for the tuberculosis patients according to the work load. Treatment would be given to the entire family at the same time, making it easier to discuss any problems encountered by either the patient or his family.

In dealing with Indian patients it is unwise to expect rigid adherence to a time schedule. Family affairs or a ceremonial rite may sometimes be expected to take precedence over medical appointments. However, since the health representative is a member of the same community he will be aware of festival schedules and can make the necessary adjustments in clinic appointments.

A four-week month should be aimed at for clinic scheduling. This insures that the clinics are always held on the same day of the week. At this monthly clinic, the Public Health Officer would be present to provide the necessary medical follow-up. Drugs can be obtained in pre-packed envelopes to cover four weeks exactly. These can be issued to the patient at this time by the attending Health Officer. Periodic home visits made by the health representative will reinforce instructions and insure that the patient and his family understand precisely what to do and are actually following medical directions.

There will always be the patient who does not take his drugs as ordered. Evidence from Madras indicates that if isoniazid and streptomycin are both given twice a week in higher than conventional doses, they can be as effective as isoniazid and para-aminosalicylic acid given daily (*Lancet*, 1963). This type of high-dosage intermittent regimen has been used in this country recently. It was used to treat a group of difficult, unreliable patients after they had undergone an initial period of treatment in a hospital. In most instances the patients came to the clinic twice a week for an injection of streptomycin and an ingestion of isoniazid. In a few instances, the public health nurse made regular twice-weekly home visits. If the patients missed a single dose of medication, they were immediately sought (Moulding, 1967). A similar method of treatment would be used for the Papago patient. The problem of locating the patient who missed an appointment would be minimized since the person administering the medications would be a neighbor. Therefore, he would be most likely to know the whereabouts of the truant patient.

PREDICTED OUTCOME

Outpatient treatment of the Papago who has tuberculosis would be the least disruptive method of treatment and control. When the patient is treated on an ambulatory, outpatient basis, family solidarity is maintained. If the patient is a head of the household, or the patriarch of a family group, he remains within the group and can continue to function as its leader and advisor.

The patient can remain at work or return to it as soon as possible. This is especially true of those Papagos whose work is performed outdoors in the fresh air and sunlight. Work is a valuable therapeutic measure; it relieves the mind and helps feed both the patient and his family.

If it becomes necessary to hospitalize the patient, allowing a family member to remain with the patient and to assist with his care also maintains the solidarity of the family unit. Furthermore, it provides strong social and human resources for emotional comfort.

Treating the medicine man as a colleague and including him in the treatment program indicates to the patient a respect for Papago beliefs and a willingness to incorporate those parts of their healing rituals that have psychotherapeutic value. The medicine man is a soul doctor who gives peace to his patients by ignoring doubt, dispelling fear, and restoring confidence. His good will can have a powerful influence in determining the degree of acceptance of hospitalization by the patient.

Village ties are also maintained by outpatient treatment. If the patient holds a political or ceremonial office he will be able to discharge his obligations without interruption of his treatment. Personal experience in caring for Papagos in a hospital setting has convinced the author that most irregular hospital discharges result from the patient's desire to attend village festivals. Sonora Catholicism is practiced by most of the inhabitants of the larger villages. The beliefs and practices of Sonora Catholics are remnants of the teaching of early Spanish missionaries, acquired either directly from padres, or through other Indians or Mexicans. There are no regular Sunday services. However, each village has its patron saint and the Saint's Day is celebrated with special ceremonies, feasting, singing, and dancing. Each village usually has two or three festivals a year. Festival responsibilities are taken seriously by the Papagos and nothing short of being totally incapacitated or being at death's door is allowed to interfere.

The use of the tribal health representative has been accepted by the Indians in those areas where he has been introduced. Members of the Indian community have been helped to better understand why it is important to seek treatment or to participate in preventive health activities. In many instances community health aides have brought patients in for treatment who had needed but resisted care, either for themselves or for their children, for days, weeks, or months.

This type of program would be flexible enough to permit modifications to fit each local situation. It would administer health care in a familiar setting, utilizing existing strengths. It would attempt to remedy weaknesses. This writer feels that such a modified flexible program would be accepted by the Papago people. Results should be apparent after a twelve month period.

Evaluation

A reduction in the number of irregular hospital discharges, fewer instances of interrupted drug therapy, and a reduction in the number of missed clinic appointments would indicate acceptance of the program. Each Indian Service clinic presently keeps a tuberculosis case file, where brief clinical notes for each known patient are kept. The records include the information mentioned. A comparison of these files at the beginning of the program and at the end of a twelve-month period for each patient included in the program would provide statistical confirmation of the acceptance or rejection of the program.

REFERENCES

Castetter, E. F., and W. H. Bell, *Pima and Papago Indian Agriculture.* Albuquerque: University of New Mexico Press, 1942.

Fontana, B. L., *Assimilative Change: A Papago Indian Case Study.* Ph.D. thesis, University of Arizona, 1960.

Fox, W., "Self-administration of Medicaments." *Bulletin International Tuberculosis Association* 32 (1962):307-31.

Hackenberg, R. A., "Aboriginal Land Use and Occupancy of the Papago Indians." Report to the U.S. Department of Justice, Lands Division, Indian Claims Section, 1964.

Hoover, J. W. "Generic Descent of the Papago Villages." *American Anthropologist*, 37 (1935):257-64.

Jones, D. J., *Human Ecology of the Papago.* Master's thesis, University of Arizona, 1962.

____. "An Analysis of Papago Communities 1900-1920." Ph.D. thesis, University of Arizona, 1969.

Kelly, W. H., *The Papago Indians of Arizona: A Population and Economic Study.* Tucson: Bureau of Ethnic Research, University of Arizona, 1963.

Moulding, T., "The Realized and Unrealized Benefits From Chemotherapy for Tuberculosis," *Public Health Reports* 82 (1967):753-58.

Sievers, M. L., "Disease Patterns Among Southwestern Indians." *Public Health Reports*, 81 (1966):1075-85.

Spicer, E. H., *Cycles of Conquest.* Tucson: University of Arizona Press, 1962.

Spicer, R. B., "People of the Desert," In *The Desert People*, edited by Alice Joseph, R. B. Spicer, and J. Chesky. Chicago: University of Chicago Press, 1949.

Tuberculosis Chemotherapy Center (Madras, India), "Intermittent Treatment of Pulmonary Tuberculosis," *Lancet* 1 (1963):1078-80.

Underhill, R. M., *Social Organization of the Papago Indians.* Columbia Contributions to Anthropology, vol. 30. New York: Columbia University Press, 1939.

____. *Papago Indian Religion.* Columbia Contributions to Anthropology, vol. 33. New York: Columbia University Press, 1946.

Waddell, J. O., *Papago Indians at Work.* Anthropological Papers of the University of Arizona, no. 12. Tucson: University of Arizona Press, 1969.

Zimmerly, D. W., "Papago Mate Selection: A Longitudinal Study," *Bulletin American Anthropological Association*, 1 (1968):153.